NATURAL IMMUNITY

NATURAL IMMUNITY

Noboru B. Muramoto

George Ohsawa Macrobiotic Foundation
Oroville, California

This book does not provide any medical diagnosis or treatment, only dietary suggestions for good health. If you are ill or on medication, consult with a physician experienced in the effects of dietary change.

Cover design: Carl Campbell of Gateway Graphics,
    San Francisco, California
Illustrations: Sheri Peterson, Oroville, California

First edition   1988

Published by the George Ohsawa Macrobiotic Foundation,
1511 Robinson Street, Oroville, California 95965

Library of Congress Catalog Card Number: 88-81555
ISBN 0-918860-48-2

Publisher's Note

Noboru Muramoto was born in Fukui Prefecture, central Japan, in November of 1920. As a young man he wanted to be a doctor of Western medicine, but he studied Oriental medicine, especially Chinese herbal medicine, instead.

After graduating from Tohoku (Imperial) University in economics, he worked in the business field. At that time he read George Ohsawa's books and studied macrobiotics. However, Ohsawa had left Japan, and he didn't meet him until a few years before Ohsawa's death in 1966. When Ohsawa died, Mr. Muramoto was elected as the head of Nippon C.I. (Centre Ignoramus), the Tokyo macrobiotic center.

In 1971 we invited Mr. Muramoto to the summer lecture tour held by the George Ohsawa Macrobiotic Foundation in the United States. His lecture at our French Meadows Summer Camp that year was his first English lecture, and it attracted many listeners. One of these people was Michel Abehsera, a New York writer, who later compiled his lecture notes taken from Muramoto's talks and created the book *Healing Ourselves*. This was later published by Avon and has been one of the best macrobiotic books as well as a favorite in the natural self-healing movement.

After finally emigrating to California in 1976, he established Asunaro, a teaching center, in Sonoma County, where he became one of the first macrobiotic consultants on the West Coast. In 1979 he relocated to southern California, where he continues to teach macrobiotics and to manufacture high quality traditional foods such as miso, umeboshi, and natural salt.

Mr. Muramoto is an avid reader gifted with a good memory and his lectures always surprise and illuminate the listener, inspiring interest in any subject. In this latest work he introduces his considerable knowledge of Western medicine and history accumulated during his more than forty years of study. However, his writing is not just an accumulation of knowledge but rather the total conclusion of his thinking after four decades of study in sickness, healing, and a macrobiotic approach to diet.

This book will appeal to macrobiotic and nonmacrobiotic readers alike and will be easy to understand because his approach is based on Western science rather than Oriental medicine.

He discusses the history of epidemics and the causes, treatment, and prevention of many illnesses, and focuses on the recent degenerative disease, AIDS. Insights are offered as to the underlying causes of AIDS and suggestions are given for strengthening the immune system naturally. Increased immunity and the prevention of any condition favorable to AIDS are the subjects here, but there is every reason to try Mr. Muramoto's approach as treatment for an existing diagnosis of AIDS or ARC.

Thanks to Matthew Piner, Jim Poggi, Sandy Rothman, and Carl Ferre for editing, and to Carl Campbell for the cover design.

Herman Aihara
President, George Ohsawa Macrobiotic Foundation

Preface

I am going to write the conclusion of this book first, as the problem is urgent and you are very busy. For the prevention of AIDS, try the following dietary suggestions for four months:

- Eat grains and vegetables.
- Do not eat meat, eggs, dairy products, or processed foods.
- No sugar, honey, syrups, or other sweets.
- Chew very well and do not overeat.

As you can see, this is just a vegetarian diet. If you already know what this means, just practice it. To know why we need such a diet and what is wrong with certain foods, please read this book. If you feel this recommendation is too strange, please read the *Dietary Goals For the United States* prepared by the Senate Select Committee on Nutrition and Human Needs (U.S. Government Printing Office, Washington, D.C., 1977), which suggested that we reduce total calorie intake; reduce meat, sugar, fat, salt, and cholesterol intake; and eat more fiber foods, such as whole grains.

Among the endorsements for the *Dietary Goals* is the following statement:

> As a nation we have come to believe that medicine and medical technology can solve our major health problems. The role of such important factors as diet in cancer and heart disease has long been obscured by the emphasis on the conquest of these diseases through the miracles of modern medicine. Treatment, not prevention, has been the order of the day.
>
> The problems can never be solved merely by more and

more medical care. The health of individuals and the health of the population is determined by a variety of biological (host), behavioral, sociocultural and environmental factors. None of these is more important than the food we eat. (*Dietary Goals,* page xix.)

If Americans had accepted the Senate Committee's recommendation, AIDS may not have spread so terribly. But unfortunately, the reaction to *Dietary Goals* was quite negative, especially from food businesses and many in the health field. In the past, so many new ideas and great discoveries have met with strong opposition; even Charles Darwin's theory of evolution took twenty years before it was widely accepted in the scientific community. Whether Darwin's theory was right or wrong, the loss of human life is not a direct result. However, if the *Dietary Goals* was correct, millions of American lives may have been unnecessarily lost during the past ten years. This includes victims of heart disease, cancer, and AIDS.

In the long run, prevention is easier than treatment or curing. However, as stated in *Dietary Goals,* we seem to have chosen treatment over prevention. Since the publication of *Dietary Goals,* about ten years have passed. Science and technology have developed more, and many new discoveries have been made. We have to go forward one step more – we cannot stay at the same stage of the *Dietary Goals.* Also, I knew it contained some mistakes.

In August, 1985 I was surprised by the cover stories of *Time* and *Newsweek* magazines. AIDS was spreading rapidly among heterosexuals. The biggest shock was that babies and children were being infected. Fear and mass hysteria have overtaken society, for AIDS is incurable. For many days I tried to think of what I could do for Americans. From my forty years of experience in natural healing, I felt that AIDS is not so mysterious a disease. I decided to write a book.

After reading the newest medical books and books on AIDS, I found that my ideas are not unusual, not opposed to modern science. I talk just about the foods we eat. Nothing more. For preventing diseases, food is most important and everyone needs to know it. Nutritional theory has undergone a big change in recent years and the new research is very good.

During the time I have been writing this book, the incidence of AIDS has been increasing about 10 percent every month. If this rate continues for five years, the total number can reach one million. Now, many AIDS patients depend on government help, paid for by taxes. How long can healthy people support so many AIDS patients? The health insurance and welfare programs may become bankrupt.

I am hoping 100 million Americans will read this book. This means almost everyone, from teenagers to the elderly, whether educated or not, rich or poor – everyone needs to know how to avoid contracting AIDS. At this time, I am unaware of any better ideas. To let everyone know is the primary purpose of this book.

Thus, I have tried to make this book easy to read and understand. Many complicated subjects have been simplified and difficult exceptional cases avoided. In these cases, specialists can advise. But the most fundamental structure, composition, and functions of the human body are not that different from person to person. Professional people might find this explanation too simplified, but perhaps in thinking about basic theory they will discover different approaches to the unknown answers.

In addition to specific suggestions for AIDS prevention, many related stories and historical examples have been included to support my opinions and provide interesting reading. These may not seem so important for the main subject, but to understand AIDS we need to know about many kinds of infections, for AIDS is not a single disease but a multiple infection.

Everyone has the right to choose which foods to eat; no one can interfere or enforce. Other people can give you suggestions or advice, and others can cook and serve for you, but whether you take it or not is still your own choice. After you've read this book, to accept my advice and practice or not is still up to you. But Nature herself is always dividing people into two groups and gives a clear answer with life or death. Watch the progression of disease carefully for the next ten years, but nothing is better than practicing before you have reason for regret.

The prevention method in this book can save the people and the government trillions of dollars. But still, I feel that even one billion dollars is nothing compared to one human life.

Contents

Introduction

We must pay attention to the simple fact that AIDS is spreading all over the world, but the number of incidences is very uneven; in some countries, no one has contracted AIDS. The highest incidence is reported in the United States, over sixty thousand as of May 1988. Next are Western European and Tropical African and Caribbean countries. High incidences are found also in Australia, New Zealand, Argentina, and the urban areas of Brazil. Mexico is our neighbor, but the reported cases are very few even though so many people are always travelling back and forth between Mexico and the United States. In some nations, diagnosis may not be accurate or exact data is unavailable. Many Asian countries have reported only a few AIDS cases, in other countries practically none. In Japan, the record is clear: thirty-six cases have been reported since 1981. Twenty-four have died and twelve are in the hospital; no Kaposi's sarcoma has been reported and the main route of transmission of the virus is said to be from imported blood. It seems that AIDS has not been passed from person to person in Japan. Among Asian descendants in the United States, surprisingly few have AIDS.

It may be true that viruses cause disease, but disease is always a complicated subject. Many co-factors have a stronger linkage to the disease than do viruses or bacteria. Epidemiologists are working to determine these linkages, such as race, sex, age, and place of residence. Many factors are being considered, including education, occupation, and personal habits like the use of tobacco and alcohol, and others. Genetic factors are sometimes emphasized, but this is wrong. AIDS is an acquired trouble. Genetic immune deficiencies

1

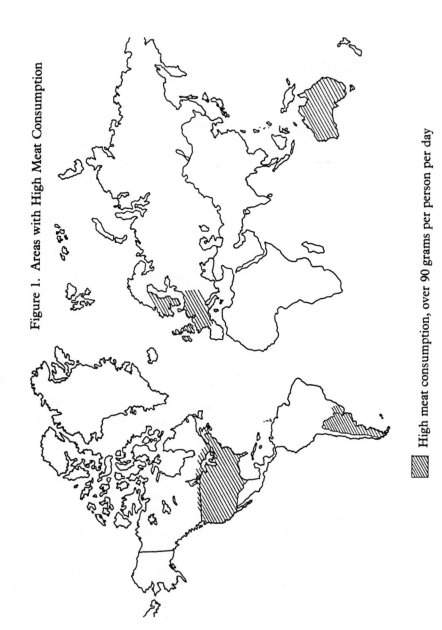

Figure 1. Areas with High Meat Consumption

High meat consumption, over 90 grams per person per day

should be treated in a different way.

To me it is clear that the most important co-factor in acquired disease is food. Finding the most suitable food for humans is the main subject of this book. Look at the world map on page 2. It is no surprise that the areas with the highest consumption of animal protein and the areas with the highest incidence of AIDS are almost exactly the same. In Tropical Africa and the Caribbean countries, sugar is another culprit. Accurate data on production and direct consumption is not available, but there is no doubt that tropical countries produce a lot of sugar, definitely in the Caribbean.

Each factor, animal food (meat) and plant food (sugar), has a specific effect on our body and health, and so American AIDS and African and Caribbean AIDS are slightly different. About 35 percent of American AIDS cases include Kaposi's sarcoma, which has a strong relationship to excess consumption of meat and animal foods, whereas only about 15 percent of the African cases include Kaposi's sarcoma. But more than 70 percent of African AIDS is related to pneumonia and tuberculosis, diseases which have a strong connection with sugar and honey.

The United States is the richest country in the world, with the most developed science, technology, education, and sanitation systems; in Africa it is the opposite, with primitive, poor, and uneducated people walking barefoot in the worst sanitary environment. But unfortunately, Africa and the United States share the highest rates of infection by the AIDS virus. What is the same in both countries? It must be the internal environment (called the *milieu interieur* by the great French physiologist Claude Bernard), which is the blood and lymphatic fluids surrounding the body cells. This environment, the blood and lymph, is made from the foods we eat. Thus, foods create either good health or disease.

In 1985 a national magazine reported that "there have been no cases of AIDS reported among a group of gay vegetarians living in New York City." This seems reasonable to me, but I don't think anyone paid any attention. The estimated United States population is 250 million, with at least 10 million people on a vegetarian diet; this proportion is about 4 percent. As of August 1987 there were about 42,000 reported cases of AIDS; if we apply the same 4 percent rate, there would be 1680 vegetarians with AIDS. But actually there are very few. Has anyone checked such an important thing? There may be 50, or maybe fewer cases. It is especially unlikely that anyone in that group had Kaposi's sarcoma. If a vegetarian contracts AIDS, it is almost always the pneumonia-tuberculosis form. Kaposi's sarcoma is also very seldom found in babies, for they do not eat meat.

My fundamental idea is that if the proportion of animal foods and plant foods is balanced in our diet, we are healthy; if we lose this balance we get sick. Food varieties and different proportions of these foods result in different physical conditions and different symptoms. A longtime enigma in the medical world has been two forms of illness arising from one kind of bacteria as the causative agent. But one form has a strong connection with excess animal foods while the other is linked with excess plant foods. If there is an excess of both plant and animal foods, there can be a mixed or border form of the disease. Excess is always bad. Even with essential foods like bread or water, excess can cause some kind of disease.

So far, no one has recovered from AIDS; many patients have died within two years. Some of the best news is that Dr. Robert Cathcart III, a renowned orthopedic surgeon in Los Altos, California, has treated AIDS successfully with large doses of vitamin C. In many of his patients, about 80 percent of the lesions from Kaposi's sarcoma have disappeared. This is great, for no one had shown any improvement but by this treatment there were such recoveries. Still, some doctors say that megadoses of vitamin C are dangerous; this is also reasonable, for we can think of vitamin C as the essence of vegetables and fruits, plant foods, which may be good balance for meat-eaters with Kaposi's but dangerous for those with *Pneumocystis carinii* pneumonia.

In the past the biggest question concerning epidemics was

the question of vulnerability to the disease, why some people contracted the disease while others did not. Now, everyone knows that those with a weakened immune system fall victim to infections. The kind of bacteria or virus does not matter, for a weak immune system is weak against any kind of infection. AIDS is no exception.

This seems obvious but still there is confusion. Many kinds of infections can be classified into two categories which have opposite characteristics. Usually a person who gets an infection from one category almost never gets an infection from the other category. This also is easy to understand. The mixed or borderline form of infections which have been increasing in recent years also make for much confusion. The reason for this increase is that people's food is becoming worse. Thus, the kinds of food that have a strong relationship with each infection, as well as each form of infection itself, are discussed in this book. The solution for AIDS can resolve all kinds of questions about infections.

Another problem is the fear and hysteria related to AIDS. This is becoming more disastrous than AIDS itself and should be conquered at the same time. People are afraid of AIDS because it is considered incurable and beyond prevention. They have no confidence in their health. When they understand that AIDS can be prevented, the fear disappears. The best and quickest way to gain this confidence is through chewing foods very well. This is not a theory or principle, but just an actual fact based on practice. Chewing makes the immune system stronger and this subject is discussed in Chapter 9. Chew one hundred times or more for each mouthful of food. If you practice, you will be surprised by the big change. Within one week your skin will look different – fresh, bright, and beautiful. Your body will not feel heavy anymore and you will be much more energetic, with no fatigue; you will feel that you have started a new life. Without doing anything else, fear will begin to disappear. You will want to continue this practice your whole life. But without actually trying this, you cannot understand. If you do not improve through this practice, the solution is to chew more.

You may think you are too busy and have no time to chew, but what is important in our life? Where is happiness without good health? You may need about one hour for a meal. I know many people who spend two hours, not for chewing but for talking. This is not bad, but now use some of this time for chewing.

Recently, I read Tatsuichiro Akizuki's book, *Nagasaki 1945* (Quartet Books, London, 1981). He was 100 percent successful in preventing three hundred patients, nurses, and workers from atomic disease. At that time, no one knew about the atomic bomb and the radiation of the bomb's explosion. He recommended that everyone eat brown rice and miso soup with a small amount of garden-fresh vegetables and seaweeds. He prohibited the eating of sugar and suggested the drinking of a salt solution. For Americans who do not have miso, there are other foods which are available and effective for AIDS prevention. His marvellous results from the application of natural foods are still largely unknown, so I have made available the most important points from his book.

In 675 A.D. a plague was spreading throughout Japan. It is difficult to determine exactly what kind of disease this was, as it is an ancient story and there are no complete records of the symptoms. But it seems the plague came from continental Asia and included high fever and a change in skin color; probably it was a form of the Black Death. Thousands were dying, but people could not do anything to stop it or slow it down. On the advice of a Buddhist priest, the emperor Temmu issued a proclamation that said, "From this day forward, do not eat beef, pork, poultry or any other meat of domestic animals. This law is effective forever." The plague was soon abated and people became healthier. The law became a Japanese tradition and was practiced for twelve hundred years. Of course, many plagues attacked them repeatedly, but still their death rate was lower than that of the Chinese or the Europeans. In the middle of the nineteenth century, the Americans arrived in Japan and trade was opened. The Americans were the first people to teach the Japanese that meat is good to eat, for it is considered to have the best nutrients. Thus, the Japanese started to eat meat.

By accident or an act of providence, I, a Japanese, came to America 130 years later, wanting to remind Americans that in order to win the battle against AIDS it is necessary to avoid eating meat.

Chapter 1

AIDS Outlook

The disease known as AIDS destroys the body's immune system, leaving the victim defenseless against a wide variety of infections. Since its discovery in mid-1981, over sixty thousand Americans have become severely ill with AIDS; more than half of them have died. Each month this number increases by the thousands. All over the world thousands more have been stricken and there seems to be no cure or end in sight. Numerous difficult questions have challenged medical researchers. Where does the disease come from? What is the cause? Is it simply one disease or is it the result of several pathogens working together? Can it be prevented by vaccines or other means? Who is at risk in contracting it? Many of these questions remain unanswered while AIDS continues to threaten many lives.

What is AIDS?

AIDS is an acronym formed by combining the first letters of the medical term used for the disease: *Acquired Immune Deficiency Syndrome*. A syndrome is a combination of many symptoms, the abnormal signs that appear in a patient. The healthy body has almost perfect protection from the causative agents of disease and can cleanse the system of harmful substances and abnormal cells produced by the body. This ability is called immunity, and the security equipment is the immune system. Acquired means obtained or gained; if someone has a special condition from his parents or ancestors, this is not acquired, but genetic. Deficiency is a shortage or lack, but in this case with the sense of something lost or failing, thus called immuno-suppression. This is the special characteristic of AIDS.

If any causative agent of disease (pathogen) enters a body with this condition, the body can be very easily defeated by it. AIDS includes many kinds of diseases, more than twenty; each of these associated diseases is called an opportunistic infection, and one sufferer often has two or more such infections. The opportunistic infections that appear most often are Kaposi's sarcoma (KS) and *Pneumocystis carinii* pneumonia (PCP). Others include *Candida albicans, Mycobacterium tuberculosis,* cryptococcosis, cytomegalovirus (CMV), herpes simplex, Burkitt's lymphoma, cryptospiridosis, and non-Hodgkin's undifferentiated lymphoma. In the near future the numbers of opportunistic infections could be in the hundreds, for any kind of pathogen can attack a weakened immune system.

These are not new infections. They are diseases that have already been well-researched and well-defined. As long as a single causative agent remains undiscovered, AIDS will be a complicated illness due to the multiplicity of infections.

Kaposi's sarcoma has been classified as a rare form of cancer and in medical history cancer has not been considered infectious or contagious, but in the last few decades many things have changed. New discoveries have shown that viruses can cause cancer, such as Burkitt's lymphoma (believed to be caused by the Epstein-Barr virus), liver cancer (related to the hepatitis B virus), and certain kinds of leukemia and lymphoma (associated with the adult T-cell leukemia virus).[1] If a virus is the cause of a disease, then this is classified as an infection and its transmissibility becomes clear.

In the past, cancer was considered a slow-growing disease, taking from ten to twenty years to develop following medical diagnosis.

But these new infectious cancers are fast-growing and fatal, such as the highly contagious Kaposi's sarcoma in AIDS cases. Thus, what causes the suppression of the immune system becomes the most important question.

What Causes AIDS?

At first, cytomegalovirus (CMV) and the Epstein-Barr virus were suspected as the causative agents of AIDS. CMV is one of the most common viruses and can be found worldwide in humans and animals. It is said that 80 percent of all Americans have the CMV antibody by the age of thirty-five or forty, so the virus is usually considered harmless. Cytomegalic inclusion disease has been seen in newborn infants before the maturing of their immune systems, and in a few adults who have had renal transplant operations. These are rather rare. But CMV, which creates immuno-suppression in the body, is often excreted in urine and saliva. In blood serum tests of a homosexual group, CMV antibodies were found in the blood of about 85 percent of those tested. But in many AIDS cases CMV did not appear as typical inclusions in the tissue lesions under microscopic examination, and could not be identified at autopsy. Thus CMV is considered a kind of causative agent.

The Epstein-Barr virus (EBV) causes mononucleosis, Burkitt's lymphoma, a type of cancer found in southern China, and an immune deficiency disorder known as a kind of herpes virus. Other viruses, such as adenoviruses, were also isolated from AIDS patients, but there is not enough evidence to show that any single one of them causes AIDS. These also are considered pathogens of opportunistic infections. Some researchers theorize from the results of bone marrow and other biopsies that *Mycobacterium tuberculosis* causes immune depression. This is not widely accepted, but it makes for more confusion.[2]

In May 1983, earlier than expected, a group of French researchers reported that they had found a probable AIDS virus, the lymphadenopathy-associated virus (LAV). At almost the same time

Dr. Robert Gallo, of the National Cancer Institute, and his colleagues discovered the human T-cell leukemia virus. But soon he understood that this virus does not cause leukemia. This virus specifically attacks the helper T-cells or T-4 lymphocytes, one type of white blood cell which plays a major role in defending the body against infections.[3] Gallo changed the name to human T-cell lymphotrophic virus (HTLV-III). Many researchers thought this was correct, but still it was not proven. Traditionally in order to establish such proof Koch's postulates must be fulfilled:

1. The organism must be observed in every case of the disease.
2. The organism must be isolated and grown in a pure culture.
3. The organism must, when inoculated into a susceptible animal, cause the disease.
4. The organism must be recovered from the experimental animal and its identity confirmed.[4]

Unfortunately, not even one of these requirements was fulfilled in testing. To be precise, almost 100 percent of the test patients should have the same virus. But actually only 30 percent of Kaposi's sarcoma patients had this HTLV-III virus while 85 percent of pre-AIDS subjects tested positive.[5]

Table 1. Isolation of HTLV-III from Patients with AIDS
and AIDS-related Conditions

Diagnosis	Number positive for HTLV-III	Number tested	Percent positive
Pre-AIDS	18	21	85.7
Clinically normal mothers of juvenile AIDS patients	3	4	75.0
Juvenile AIDS	3	8	37.5
Adult AIDS with Kaposi's sarcoma	13	43	30.2
Adult AIDS with opportunistic infections	10	21	47.6
Clinically normal homosexual donors	1	22	4.5
Clinically normal heterosexual donors	0	115	0

The AIDS virus is still not definitely determined. Look carefully at the future research.

More Than One Kind of Microbe

Some researchers speculate that HTLV-III causes immuno-suppression and then leaves the body; a secondary virus then utilizes this favorable condition and causes an opportunistic infection such as Kaposi's sarcoma or PCP. This idea is interesting, but if the virus has left the body, the patient could recover from the immune deficiency. However, this does not happen. Probably HTLV-III is one of the causative agents of AIDS, followed by HTLV-II and HTLV-IV. Cytomegalovirus and some other herpes viruses also cause immuno-suppression and are considered causative agents of AIDS. If this is true, you can see how complicated AIDS can be.

In the past, it has been considered that one disease is caused by one kind of microbe – tuberculosis by *Mycobacterium tuberculosis,* syphilis by *Treponema pallidum.* But now, with AIDS, two or more different microbes work together in a complex way. This is said to be a new form of disease, but whether this is exactly new is questionable. A long time ago leprosy and tuberculosis patients often died from attacks by secondary pathogens; also pneumonia bacteria killed many flu patients. These examples are well known.

Another difficulty in AIDS research is that test animals have not been successfully inoculated with the HTLV-III virus. AIDS is still an exclusively human disease. African green monkeys are assumed to be the original hosts of the AIDS virus, but they do not contract the disease. For them it seems to be harmless. Some reports have indicated that researchers have succeeded in inoculating chimpanzees with the AIDS virus; some symptoms similar to AIDS appeared, but in these cases there was no evidence that either KS or PCP occurred.[6] If a good vaccine or drug were made, there is no way to test it on animals. Even if someone succeeded with animal tests, a long incubation period (from one to seven years) would be needed for results. The effectiveness of such vaccines and drugs, the proper dosages, the safety factors, the side effects, the toxic reactions – all these should be tested. The next step would be human testing. Then it would be at least ten years before we could expect to have a good vaccine, and by then the cases could surpass twenty-two million. If many kinds of viruses cause AIDS, then many kinds of vaccines are needed and the time required to conquer AIDS will be even greater. Also, a vaccine has no power to reverse the disease process; it can only work towards prevention.

Routes of Transmission

At first AIDS appeared among homosexual men and was called the gay plague. The next groups affected were drug abusers and hemophiliacs who received blood transfusions. Most frightening of all was the appearance of AIDS in infants whose mothers were infected. No longer the gay plague, AIDS is clearly a bloodborne disease (spread through blood and body fluids), even though people still refer to it as a sexually transmitted disease.

Insect vectors are another possible source of transmission. This may be the case in Belle Glade, Florida, a small sugar-producing town near Palm Beach that has been called a "world-class ghetto" and the "AIDS capital of the world." From 1982 to August of 1985, this town of twenty thousand has reported forty-six cases of AIDS, about three times the per capita incidence in New York or San Francisco. Twenty-two, or almost half, of these victims do not fall into any of the high risk categories.[7] One theory on this pattern relates to the abnormally large numbers of mosquitoes breeding in the unsanitary conditions of Belle Glade, but this is unlikely since AIDS does not follow any of the usual patterns of diseases spread by mosquitoes, such as malaria (bacterial), yellow fever, or some kinds of encephalitis (viral). Researchers speculate that mosquitoes do not transport a sufficient quantity of blood and virus to pose any danger, but this still remains a slight possibility. The spread of AIDS by flea, tick, or other insect bites, as in bubonic plague, is a possibility that has not been fully studied.

As of 1985 in the United States there were more than eight hundred cases of AIDS with unknown sources of transmission.

AIDS in Africa

In African countries, where AIDS is widespread, incidences of PCP (*Pneumocystis carinii* pneumonia) are higher than those of Kaposi's sarcoma. When one member of a family has been infected with AIDS, the incidence of other family members getting AIDS triples, even where sexual relations with the infected person are not involved. Men and women contract AIDS almost equally and AIDS among children is very common. In Haiti AIDS is also accompanied by PCP and tuberculosis as opportunistic infections.

Before the epidemic of AIDS, PCP was rather rare. It is a virulent form of pneumonia which affects mainly newborn infants whose immune systems are not yet developed. PCP is believed to be caused by a protozoa-like microorganism carried through the air via the respiratory system. A few researchers believe that the microbes are carried by insects. Among adults, PCP affects the weakened elderly, the extremely ill, and those who have had kidney transplants.[8]

Tuberculosis and pneumonia are generally believed to be airborne diseases. No one would say that they are sexually transmitted. But in African and Haitian AIDS, it seems too early to say that the disease is never spread by insect bites or through the air. I am not trying to emphasize controversial opinion. I just want to say that as long as the AIDS problem concerns human life, our course should be absolutely safe. Even a tiny mistake cannot be allowed. At this point, without any further checking, to say AIDS is a sexually transmitted disease is a mistake, even if the factors of drug abuse and blood transfusion are added.

Exposed and Infected

It would be good to find out how contagious AIDS is compared with other epidemic diseases. Probably the most familiar one is measles. Almost every adult has experienced this disease or was vaccinated during childhood and has immunity to it. So, measles is considered a children's disease. A sudden outbreak usually occurs every three or four years, attacking almost the entire population in crowded areas. At that time previously uninfected children are infected. This often happens at the opening of primary school or kindergarten. The measles virus is transmitted through the air, so it quickly spreads everywhere. But the symptoms are not severe and the death rate is only about one in ten thousand or .01 percent. In rural areas and isolated places such as islands, children can grow up without being infected. Once the virus invades these areas, the destruction is disastrous for the adult population. The symptoms are more severe and highly fatal. It is better to have been infected early. To clarify: *exposed* means that the population has the opportunity to contract the disease; *infected* means that the causative agent of the disease has already entered the bloodstream.

Another epidemic is the flu. In 1918 an influenza known as the Spanish Flu spread all over the world. Six hundred million people got this disease and twenty-three million died. Of those exposed, 70 percent became infected and developed full-blown symptoms and about 4 percent of those afflicted died. To be exact, this percentage includes deaths from secondary attacks by pneumonia.

In the case of AIDS, researchers guess that between 2 and 3 million Americans have been exposed to the AIDS virus and are carriers. If we compare this figure with the entire population of 250 million, the percentage is minimal – about 1 percent. The number of those who have full-blown AIDS compared with the number of those infected is 1 percent or less (only .01 percent of the total population). The AIDS virus is not highly contagious.

But if we look at the death rate, already about thirty-four thousand have died and others have almost no hope of recovery. Within an average eighteen-month period, 100 percent of the victims seem to be dying. Among the many epidemics in the history of

Figure 2. Comparisons of Degenerative Diseases

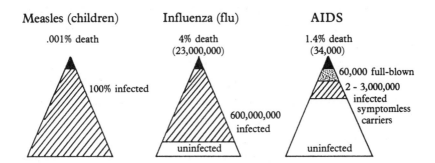

disease, this death rate is very unusual. There are only a few we can compare it with; one of these rare diseases is rabies.

Rabies is a type of encephalitis caused by a virus which is transmitted by a rabid animal bite, in the case of humans usually from a dog. Only a few cases of bites from other animals, such as bats, cats, wolves, or others have been reported. Written records concerning rabies date back to ancient Greece, so it is not a new disease. By the eighteenth century rabies had spread all over Europe and had become one of the most feared epidemics. Terrified people killed millions of healthy dogs, because almost 100 percent of the victims died and there was no means of prevention or cure. The incubation period for rabies is approximately one to three months, depending on the location of the bite on the body. For example, if the bite was on the leg, it would be about fifty days; if on the trunk, forty days; on the head, twenty days. For humans the most dangerous time was the incubation period in newly-infected dogs; the dogs looked healthy and friendly, but they would bite at the slightest provocation. After the onset of symptoms, patients died within several days. Surely rabies was a terrible disease, given that the victim was exposed, infected, and died in such short order. The disease process of AIDS is one hundred times slower than that of rabies. The rabies virus resembles AIDS HIV (human immunodeficiency virus, the new name for HTLV-III) in that it is considered to be a retrovirus (a group of viruses that have RNA instead of DNA inside the genes) and therefore belongs to the same category. However, in the case of AIDS, it is often unclear as to when the person was exposed to the virus.

Louis Pasteur succeeded in making a new vaccine for rabies, but even with a good vaccine it was difficult to cure all the patients. Some died and the deaths were blamed on the vaccine. In France, the threat of lawsuits and violent conflicts broke out at the Academy of Medicine and made their way into the Chamber of Deputies and into the political journals. In England an official commission investigated Pasteur's work and confirmed the positive results of his treatments.[10] Experience later showed that Pasteur's critics were entirely wrong. Louis Pasteur became very famous and respected.

If the AIDS virus came from the African green monkey, we are fortunate not to have many of them in this world. However, AIDS is transmitted only from human to human. What is the percent of infection in relation to the numbers of people exposed? There is no way to find out, since our sex lives are private. Here is one estimate written by a San Francisco Bay Area reporter in June 1983: "If AIDS is indeed sexually transmitted, why have there been so few cases? I say few because if an estimated 20 million gays have an estimated 200 'sexual contacts' per year, this means that in 4 and a half years we have seen 1279 AIDS cases in 4 billion contacts."[11] Many reports indicate that some people who had sexual relationships with full-blown AIDS patients did not develop any AIDS symptoms, even after many years.

High-risk and Low-risk Groups

Most plagues and epidemics begin in large cities. AIDS is no exception. New York, San Francisco, Los Angeles, and other urban areas are the most dangerous places for contracting the disease.

Rural areas are safer and mountain regions are the safest.

Recently, most of the AIDS research has been concentrated on the high-risk group. This is good and many things became clear, but not much discussion has focused on the low-risk group.

Strangely, about 90 percent of all AIDS victims are men; the remaining 10 percent are women. Homosexuals and bisexuals are the largest group numerically, about 70 percent; drug abusers make up about 17 percent; blood recipients account for less than 1 percent. Ninety percent of the victims are between twenty and forty-nine years of age. Older people and children are safer. Broken down according to racial and ethnic groups, 59 percent are whites, 26 percent blacks, and 14 percent of Hispanic origin. Researchers James R. Allen and James W. Curran offer this interesting statistic:

> Surprisingly, of the first 4,000 patients with AIDS, only 14 were Asians or members of other ethnic groups. . . . Compared with the incidence rates of AIDS in other racial groups, the incidence rate in Asians in the United States is considerably lower than would have been predicted statistically, suggesting that risk factors for exposure to the causative virus or susceptibility factors for disease may be lower in this group.[12]

Hispanics are extremely high on the list, since many Haitians have had AIDS, but the percentage of descendants of Asians is very low. Checking Curran and Allen for details, it is even more surprising, for among these fourteen cases, six were homosexuals, one was a drug user, four had received blood transfusions, and three were unknown. The majority of Asian peoples are grain-eaters and therefore in the low-risk group for AIDS. American vegetarians are also in the low-risk group.

In 1984 Dr. Ann Hardy of the Centers for Disease Control made the following predictions in regard to the numbers of AIDS cases:[13]

Table 2. AIDS Cases

	AIDS Cases			People Infected (estimated)	
Year	Calendar	Cumulative	Year	Calendar	Cumulative
1981	239	296	1978	2,500	3,000
1982	665	961	1979	7,000	10,000
1983	1,540	2,501	1980	15,000	25,000
1984	4,499	7,100	1981	45,000	70,000
1985 (est.)	8,500	15,600	1982	85,000	155,000
1986 (est.)	15,000	30,600	1983	150,000	305,000
1987 (est.)	27,000	57,000	1984	270,000	575,000

These figures are surprisingly accurate, but too conservative. Case numbers are actually doubling every year. If this rate continues to double, the numbers would be as follows:

Table 3. AIDS Projections

Year	White	Black	Asian
1984	4,200	1,800	14
1985	8,400	3,600	28
1986	16,800	7,200	56
1987	33,600	14,400	112
1988	67,200	28,800	224
1989	134,400	57,600	448
1990	268,800	105,200	896
1991	537,600	310,400	1,792
1992	1,075,200	620,800	3,584
1993	2,150,400	1,241,600	7,168
1994	4,300,800	2,483,200	14,336
1995	8,601,600	4,966,400	28,672
1996	17,203,200	9,932,800	57,344
1997	34,406,400	19,805,600	114,688
1998	78,812,800	38,731,200	229,376
1999	157,625,600	77,462,400	458,742
2000	315,250,200	154,934,800	917,484
Projections based on 1986 U.S. population:	200,000,000	40,000,000	3,000,000

Before the end of the year 2000 the numbers of AIDS victims will exceed the present population. Only Asian people will survive. Is this Darwin's law of natural selection at work?

I don't think that such a thing will actually happen. Such calculations are a kind of game based on assumptions. In the plagues of the past, eventually the disease would run its course and stop on its own, for not everyone has a weak immune system. Also, in such situations, human intelligence can find ways of preventing and stopping the spread of the disease. One example was simply to exile the sick from cities and society. Until the Middle Ages they were often just banished. Then, isolation and quarantine systems developed. At the time of the London plague in 1665, sick people were locked up in their homes under guard and front doors were painted with huge red crosses. To protect the general public, this was considered to be the best possible way. In today's world, such a policy would be considered inhumane and could not be enacted.

In Mexico there are not many cases of AIDS. But if Mexican people come to the United States, they learn the dietary pattern from whites and blacks, and they develop the same problems as other Americans. Asian descendants tend more to continue the dietary patterns of their mother countries.

Proper food can prevent many kinds of diseases. If people can achieve better health through dietary change, then isolation and quarantine are not necessary. Again, AIDS is not highly contagious. And it is not good to wait for effective drugs or vaccines because they will be too late. I am not saying that Asian people are eating the best food, but still they are doing better than others. We have to find out what is good and what is wrong with each of the important foods in our daily lives.

Early Warnings of AIDS and ARC

During the long incubation period of AIDS there are some signs before the actual symptoms appear. These important signs are known as prodromes, one or more of which may emerge. They are listed here in the approximate order of their appearance:

1. Fatigue and malaise
2. Weight loss
3. Fever and chills
4. Headache and confusion
5. Shortness of breath, night sweating
6. Severe muscle aches and/or sore throat
7. Swollen lymph nodes (glands)
8. Abnormal bleeding
9. Skin rashes
10. Persistent diarrhea
11. Lesions in the mouth, nose, or anus[14]

Nothing is new or unusual within the first seven. Hundreds of kinds of diseases carry similar signs – the common cold, flu, tuberculosis, hepatitis, rheumatism, pyelonephritis. How does one know if these signs are signaling AIDS?

Whatever the cause of these signals, care should be taken at this stage. What should you do? Take aspirin, antibiotics, or some other drug? No. Taking medications or drugs is one of the major reasons why some people have weakened immune systems. New medical research shows that all such treatments have some detrimental effects on the body.

The first sign, fatigue, has the most important meaning. Usually fatigue or tiredness comes from overworking. Heavy physical labor, intensive training, and other kinds of hard work create fatigue, but after a good night's sleep or two or three days' rest, it ends. If your recovery is not good, this is a problem. The easiest way to find out is at waking time in the morning. If you can get up immediately, this is good, but if you want to stay in bed more, then this is chronic fatigue and your diet is not good.

If the disease advances, signs 8 through 11 will appear. As the virus increases in the body, the development of the disease approaches the state known as the AIDS Related Complex (ARC). Weight loss may be greater than 10 percent of body weight (or fifteen pounds) and the fever may become persistent, but life-threatening infections do not yet appear. At this stage it is still difficult to determine if the person has AIDS. A certain percentage of people with ARC develop full-blown AIDS. Some researchers claim that this percentage is large, but fortunately, right now, it is lower than expected, indicating strong resistance to the AIDS virus.

Once the disease progresses beyond these early prodromes into full-blown AIDS, recovery is almost hopeless. Antibiotics, chemotherapies, radiation treatments, interferons, interleukins – all kinds of orthodox treatments may be applied, but none of them seem to help.[15] AIDS patients often try other treatments, such as homeopathic medicine, chiropractic, acupuncture, psychotherapies, palm healing, and others. Sometimes improvement is shown, a decrease or disappearance of Kaposi's sarcoma, or a prolonged life span from four to five years instead of the less-than-two-year average, but not a complete recovery. Sooner or later almost 100 percent of AIDS patients die.

Here is an interesting report related to the early prodromes. As reported by Dr. James I. Slaff, in *Lancet,* a British medical journal, a nurse accidentally pricked herself with a needle that had been used on an AIDS patient, actually injecting a small amount of the infected blood into her bloodstream. Thirteen days after the accident she reported a severe "flu-like" illness which was characterized by headache, a mild sore throat, muscle ache, and facial pains. On the seventeenth day a rash appeared on her chest and trunk. The rash lasted for one week during which time it spread to the neck and face. Fever, general depression, and swollen glands accompanied these reactions. Within one month of the accident all these signs and symptoms had receded and disappeared. She recovered. Dr. Slaff comments: "This suggests with respect to infected blood a 'critical mass' of contagion must be injected." But anyone who has studied microbiology for even one hour knows that this does not make sense. Microbes can increase very rapidly if they have enough nutrition and a suitable environment. Many kinds of bacteria can multiply at an astounding rate. A few bacteria can become trillions in one day, and viruses can increase a hundred times faster than bacteria. Simply, we have to think that the nurse's immune system worked properly.

We know also that the majority of the homosexual population has not contracted AIDS. Extreme fear of AIDS is unnecessary.

Fear and Hysteria

Since AIDS is considered incurable, fear and mass hysteria have appeared, shaking the whole society. Even in hospitals some patients have been treated like lepers. In New York, some under-takers have refused to embalm the remains of AIDS patients; an ambulance refused to transport a patient. In the schools, parents are in conflict with each other about whether children infected with AIDS should be in the classroom.

Is such discrimination right? Is quarantine necessary? There is much discussion but no conclusions. If many people have weak immune systems, a quarantine might be good, but it would be impossible to isolate two to three million virus carriers (the esti-mated number of those exposed).

Other problems have arisen in regard to blood tests. Some deve-loped AIDS after receiving blood transfusions. This discovery resulted in blood testing on all stored blood and blood donors. One test is called ELISA, meaning "enzyme-linked immunosorbent assay" test; another is the western blot test. All blood that does not pass these tests is removed. Since the blood screening tests have been applied, the number of bad accidents has decreased dramati-cally; this was very successful but still it seems that it is not perfect. Some exceptional cases have occurred, calling the blood tests into question.

To protect healthy people from virus carriers, it would be good to test each person of the entire population, but there is not enough equipment, facilities, or technicians, so it can only be given to special high-risk groups.

It is difficult to test for the AIDS virus itself. The ELISA test only tests for an antibody of the AIDS virus. It should be 100 percent accurate, but about 5 percent of error seems inevitable. The reason for the mistakes is not well understood.

Some mistakes have been made in the testing itself; some full-blown AIDS patients have tested negative. Some who tested positive the first time have tested negative the second. It would not be good to force the public to take such inaccurate tests. Even if the blood test were more accurate, it would be almost useless as a protective measure for the general public because the results would be kept secret. AIDS discrimination is prohibited by law, but individuals are actually discriminated against.

Also, some of the AIDS virus carriers will never get AIDS in their lives because they are protected by strong antibodies as we saw in the case of measles. These people are stronger than unexposed people. An example is the prevalence of the Epstein-Barr virus which is believed to be carried in about 80 percent of the U.S. population. The carriers themselves almost never get mononucleosis, but they can pass the virus on to others.

The point of view of an AIDS patient is different from that of the public. In its most extreme expression some patients do not care whether they spread the disease or not. They just want to enjoy the two years of life that may be left to them. They want to eat their favorite foods and have sex as they choose, whether their partners are thereby infected or not. Some patients have begun to refuse their blood tests.

Plagues are public problems; the government and society as a whole try to keep them from spreading. But disease is personal. If you get sick, the pain, the sufferings, and all that goes with it belong to you. No one can take your place and experience your pain or suffering. It is said that AIDS is the only disease which is politically protected. Tuberculosis, cancer, and other patients have never been helped like AIDS patients. But as the number of patients increases, the public help will be exhausted and further help cannot be expected. Thus, it is good to establish protective measures by yourself.

When it comes to food and what you eat, you are absolutely free. Everything is your choice. No one can force any food on you; your mind, your mouth, or your throat can refuse such undesired food. Since foods create the ability of immuno-suppression, you are responsible for your disease. You are also responsible for your cure, which you can bring about by changing your diet. I can give you good advice, but only you can accept it; whether or not you practice is up to you.

Chapter 2

Plagues and Epidemics

History repeats itself. Once plagues were thought to be almost conquered, but now we have AIDS and it is considered a modern plague. It may be useful to examine plagues and afflictions of the past and how they were dealt with.

The past records show that humanity has repeatedly suffered from widespread diseases: leprosy, smallpox, typhoid, pestis, eruptive fever, cholera, malaria, tuberculosis, various types of influenza, etc. It is hard to say which was the worst epidemic since each was terrible in its own right. Before our ancestors became aware of the causes and successful treatments of these diseases, fatalities were very high. Over time our knowledge has grown, enabling us to avoid the majority of these diseases; we know what microbes cause them, how they are transmitted, how they can be prevented, and, with the discovery of antibiotics and other treatments, how they can be abated and cured.

AIDS has become a kind of plague or epidemic in many ways similar to the terrible afflictions of the Middle Ages. The misconceptions, fears, and accusations demonstrate that people do not really understand the disease. Different diseases of the past can teach us how to deal sanely with AIDS or any new infectious diseases. Leprosy, tuberculosis, and pestis are particularly useful because of their slight similarity to AIDS. It is interesting that each of these diseases follows the pattern noted in the Introduction: they appear in two forms even though there is just one kind of bacteria. The virus which causes AIDS is not just one kind, but still we can see two typical forms of disease.

In comparing diseases the first thing to look at is the way they are transmitted: by air, water, or blood/body fluids. Influenza, pneumonia, tuberculosis, measles, and mumps are all spread by airborne microorganisms. These diseases spread very extensively and rapidly, since it is nearly impossible to monitor the air we breathe or to control the way the wind blows. The microorganisms are taken in directly through the respiratory organs and are spread by sneezing, breathing on foods, and so on. The bacteria which cause typhoid, cholera, and dysentery come from contaminated water. AIDS, gonorrhea, syphilis, leprosy, and pestis are diseases which are spread only by direct contact of blood and certain other body fluids such as semen and mucus which contain microbes, depending on the specific pathogen. As mentioned in the last chapter, the unusual thing about AIDS is that the opportunistic diseases which attack the immuno-suppressed condition become the killers. Most of these are spread through the air as in the cases of *Pneumocystis carinii* pneumonia (PCP) and *Mycobacterium* tuberculosis. It is not clear how Kaposi's sarcoma is transmitted, since it is considered a cancer and as such is categorized as a medical unknown.

Leprosy

Leprosy is probably the best known of the ancient diseases. Almost every culture and country of the world has a long history of this disease. For centuries its cause was unknown and there was no treatment. As an extremely ugly-looking and incurable disease it was universally considered a divine punishment. There was great fear of its spreading and those with the disease were exiled to leper colonies, long known as dreaded places of great suffering.

Although leprosy was known among the ancient Hebrews,

Greeks, and Romans, the disease did not appear in Northern Europe until the sixth century. At this time the ancient Roman Empire had collapsed completely. For the Europeans, the largest predators were the Romans who took all the good things which others produced. When the Europeans took back their power, they acquired a new disease without knowing the reason. But still leprosy was not prevalent until the time of the Crusades. Records show that the Western crusade warriors contracted leprosy in Jerusalem, but leprosy is a slow-growing disease with an incubation period of two to seven and often up to ten years. Even for the patient it is difficult to recognize when and where exposure to the bacteria occurred. So, much of the leprosy associated with the Crusades may actually have been syphilis.

In Europe prior to 1500, leprosy was considered highly contagious and was associated with sexual contact. We can imagine that the leprosy bacteria can be transmitted easily through sexual contacts, but this was not the main route of the transmission. Repeated direct contacts with patients gave opportunities to contact the bacteria. Still the incidence of leposy was rather low, probably less than one percent of the population even at the peak of the epidemic, and it was not highly contagious. Many lepers died from other infections. Women especially had stronger resistance for this disease. In the leprosy hospitals, doctors sometimes fell to this disease, but almost no women nurses got the disease, a phenomenon also found with Kaposi's sarcoma.

In 1873 the Norwegian physician Gerhard H. A. Hansen (1841-1912) discovered the bacteria that causes leprosy, *Mycobacterium leprae.* This was the first bacillus to be associated with a chronic human disease. Because of the great social stigma associated with the word leprosy, the disease has since been called Hansen's disease to help avoid the negative connotations of uncleanliness, divine punishment, and hereditary transmission.

The disease is similar to AIDS in the way it slowly and insidiously develops without the victim's awareness. Even after the symptoms appear, it continues to progress at a slow pace, lasting anywhere from ten to twenty years in a long-lived patient. This is different from AIDS. One form of leprosy causes the whole body to appear to decay; the victim looks hideous, even monstrous. This is the typical leprosy known as lepromatous or cutaneous leprosy.

There is another form of the same disease, caused by the same *Mycobacterium*, creating an entirely different appearance in the patient. This variety is known as tuberculoid leprosy. For some reason, in this form the disease mainly attacks the nervous system. First there appear patches of discolored skin that lose sensation to physical stimuli. Then the victim loses weight and becomes extremely weak and thin as the muscles all over the body lose sensation and function, followed by a shrinkage or atrophy of the muscle tissue. If the disease progresses, further nerve damage causes crippling deformities. Although disfigurement remains for one's whole life, this second form neither produces the hideousness of lepromatous leprosy nor is it as deadly. Often, all bacteria disappear and the patient recovers. It is rarely contagious. Intermediate, mixed forms of the two types also occur and are referred to as borderline or mixed leprosy.

Leprosy is still a problem in humid, tropical, or subtropical areas, mainly in parts of Asia, India, Central Africa, South America, the Caribbean, and the Pacific Islands. There are probably ten million or more victims throughout the world.

Leprosy is our first example of two forms of a disease from the same pathogen.

Tuberculosis – The Beautiful Disease

As leprosy decreased, tuberculosis increased throughout Europe. In the case of tuberculosis, or consumption, patients lose weight and become rather emaciated, but the skin can become very beautiful in contrast to the hideous appearance of the leper. (However, some leprosy patients also have very beautiful skin in the early stages of the disease.) Tuberculosis was most often found among frail, intellectual types of people in urban areas and among factory workers, and much less often in rural areas or among peasants.

Tuberculosis is characterized by a long incubation period; again, this is similar to the *Pneumocystis carinii* pneumonia form of AIDS. The patient develops a cough and then has a low fever in the afternoons. This is followed by physical exhaustion, bed sweating, weight loss, expulsion of blood and mucus from the bronchia, and, finally, vomiting of blood from the lungs.

In the United States, a 618 per 100,000 mortality rate was reported in Philadelphia in 1845.[1] The name tuberculosis comes from the tiny, grey, nodule-like cheesy tubercles (lesions) produced by the *Mycobacterium tuberculosis* that usually attack and take form in the lungs. Note that leprosy comes from the same genus, *Mycobacterium*. Bone marrow biopsies from AIDS patients reveal a high incidence of *Mycobacterium* infection in the bone. Today more than half of the Haitian AIDS victims have tuberculosis as an opportunistic infection.

As with leprosy, there is a second form of tuberculosis (tuberculosis verrucous or tuberculosis papulonecrotic, commonly called warty tuberculosis) which appears to be caused by the same bacterium. This version of the disease may affect any number of organs other than the lungs, including the lymph nodes, the genitals, and the kidneys, and usually appears more like leprosy with the formation of wart-like pimples on the surface of the skin.

The rate of infection by tuberculosis has been steadily declining since the 1950s, but is now making a dramatic comeback, most likely as a result of the AIDS epidemic. Reports of an increase in tuberculosis all over the world, especially in Africa and the Caribbean countries where AIDS is also very prevalent, may indicate that a global tuberculosis problem is beginning again. The tuberculosis bacteria are highly contagious. However, they enter the body of a healthy individual and remain dormant and harmless unless that individual's immune system is weakened. As more people get AIDS, more are also likely to develop tuberculosis, infecting more people and so on.

Mycobacterium avium is a kind of tuberculosis bacteria which causes disease in birds, but researchers have found this bacteria in bone marrow biopsies of many AIDS patients. Tuberculosis bacteria are floating around in the air everywhere.

Leprosy, Tuberculosis, and Sex

Leprosy provides an example that of the body's organs the sex organs are among the strongest and most disease resistant. Inside the leper colonies and hospitals, patients were free to do whatever they pleased. There are documented cases of quarantined lepers who married and had disease-free children. The parents' bodies were almost completely decayed, but still they could produce perfectly healthy babies. The sex organs and the ability of the human organism to reproduce is powerful indeed. The babies were healthy because the placenta somehow filtered out the bacteria, while in certain viral diseases, such as AIDS, it cannot, so the baby becomes infected.

Tuberculosis patients also had perfectly healthy children. With tuberculosis, patients would become so thin that they would often eat large amounts of meat in an attempt to gain weight and strength. This excessive consumption of meat gave them an excessively heightened sexual desire. The sexual activity left them more weakened and exhausted, so they ate more meat and were driven to more sex, and so on. But excessive consumption of meat was not the real root of their problem. It was actually sugar.

Sugar robs the body of calcium and protein as well as other minerals and nutrients. The body then takes protein and minerals from itself in order to compensate for this loss and to keep the composition of the blood correct. In the case of tuberculosis it is the muscles and lung tissues that mainly lose protein, leaving the lungs vulnerable to bacteria. This initiates a slow, degenerative process that is helped along by the tuberculosis bacteria. Eating more meat compensates for protein loss but makes the blood more acidic and results in kidney malfunction, a condition which causes excess water to be released through the skin; this is the bed sweating found among tuberculosis patients. Calcium injections were once considered effective, but it was the discovery and use of antibiotics that accounted for the conquest of tuberculosis and the rapid decrease in the number of its victims.

Pestis – The Biggest Killer

Probably the best known of all the plagues and the biggest killer was pestis (also called La Peste, the Black Death, Bubonic Plague, Oriental Plague – the different names come from outbreaks of the disease throughout history in various forms). The abundant information about this disease contributes to our understanding of AIDS and the probable development of other infectious diseases in the future. One of the oldest accounts comes from the Old Testament.

> For death had filled the city with panic; God's hand was heavy upon it. (I Samuel 5:11-12.) They said, "If you return the ark of the God of Israel, do not send it away empty, but by all means send a guilt offering to him. Then you will be healed, and you will know why his hand has not been lifted from you." The Philistines asked, "What guilt offering should we send to him?" They replied, "Five gold tumors and five gold rats, according to the number of Philistine rulers, because the same plague has struck you and your rulers." (I Samuel 6:3-4)

Historians approximate the date of this entry to be around the eleventh century B.C. There are numerous diseases that produce symptoms of swollen lymph nodes, especially in the area of the groin, but the mention of rats is most interesting. Since the discovery in the late 1800s of the bacillus *Pasteurella pestis* (the new name is *Yersinia pestis*), it has been known that the disease was caused by bacteria carried by black rats. Fleas would bite the infected rats and then bite humans. This is the main route of this bacteria's transmission.

The most devastating recorded outbreak of the plague occurred during the mid-1300s in Europe. In approximately five years' time it claimed over twenty-five million lives and is usually referred to as the Black Death. Historical records indicate that the plague was actually an outcome of events that had occurred a few decades earlier in Asia.

In 1212 A.D. Mongolia invaded China, destroying much of the Chinese culture and establishing a new empire that would eventually develop into the largest country ever. The book *The History of Yuan* (Yuan was the Mongol Empire) states that in 1334 ". . . there were disastrous floods and great hordes of grasshoppers attacked the farmland. People suffered famine and ate each other. A plague broke out and killed five million people." In the same year the people were suffering from a shortage of salt because of floods washing out the salt beds. The price of salt was driven up and the Mongolian government took advantage of the situation by adopting a salt monopoly. The Chinese writer's description is short, simple, and powerful. It is not clear whether he is saying that cannibalism caused the plague or if he just wanted to express the severity of the starvation, but it is easy to believe that the people ate anything edible, including small animals like rats, earthworms, or whatever.

The Yuan period is a kind of Dark Age in Chinese history and not many other records have survived. Longtime Asian historians say that five million people were killed. This is probably overstated, but still only amounts to 7 percent of the Chinese population at that time. Compared to the numbers from European records, 7 percent is much lower than the European's 25 percent. By the early 1300s Europeans had already emerged from the Dark Ages. Northern Italian cities such as Venice, Bologna, and Florence were enjoying great prosperity as the trading and cultural centers of Europe. Marco Polo had returned from China in 1295. Tremendous amounts of merchandise were coming from Arabia, Africa, India, and now China, by both land and sea. The well-known Silk Road was the trade route used from China to Rome by way of Syria. But this road also became a rat- and flea-infested route, the Peste Road. At that time people were simply unaware of what devastation this added cargo of rats would bring.

Although many historical records point to different origins such as Egypt, Ethiopia, or Central Asia, an Arabian named Ibn Khatima, wrote in a Spanish text that the disease came from China, the eastern edge of the world. Before the great plague swept the European continent it was preceded by a number of strange natural disasters and signs. In 1337 hordes of grasshoppers appeared; in 1341 a hurricane struck Italy, leaving grasshoppers covering the beaches. A putrid smell was spread by the wind to the surrounding cities and countrysides. Also, a mysterious and terrible smell was reported to have come from the East.

European records state that pestis occurred first in 1346 in the Caucasus and Crimean areas of Turkey and in northern Persia. Then in 1347 it hit Sicily and Sardinia; Italy, France, and Spain in 1348; Germany and England in 1349; Denmark in 1350; Russia in 1351. Curiously it passed over Poland. A great puzzlement to many historians and medical researchers, the fact that Poland was spared is relatively easy to understand. Under the Peasant King, Casimir III, the Polish people were poor and could not afford to eat much meat. This was in contrast to the wealth and dietary habits of much of the rest of Europe at that time.

According to the great Byzantine historian, Procopius, in his book *The Persian Wars,* an earlier outbreak of the plague occurred during the Dark Ages in 540 A.D. in Egypt and spread from there to Europe. It was known as Justinian's plague and may have been larger than the disaster of the fourteenth century, but records are incomplete in Western Europe. Prior to this outbreak of pestis there was also an infestation of grasshoppers, first in northern Africa and later in Italy. Procopius states that for many days the sky became dark from the hordes of insects, leaving the farmlands and countryside barren of vegetation. After that time the plague recurred in small waves at intervals about fifteen years apart lasting for about two hundred years in Europe. The strange thing is that grasshoppers have been recently increasing in the northwestern part of the United States. Is this a coincidence?

> 540-750 A.D.: The Justinian plague was long-lasting and recurring with an estimated one hundred million deaths.
>
> 1034: Slow-moving plague because transportation and trade had not yet developed.
>
> 1348-1351: The Black Death claimed about a quarter of the population of Europe, twenty-five million; in some cases two-thirds to three-fourths of a given region perished.
>
> 1662-1666: The Great Plague of London occurred in 1664-1665, taking about seventy thousand lives; many other European countries were afflicted.
>
> 1980-?: Will pestis or something similar strike the West again?

As you can see, beginning in 750, pestis attacked Western civilization in Europe in big waves regularly at intervals of about 310 years. The intervals of the above dates may be just coincidental, but history and nature do have patterns; it would be wise to pay attention in order to prevent further disasters. Pestis, AIDS, and other deadly infectious diseases can be prevented by understanding the nature of the microbe kingdom and by strengthening our immune systems against their attack.

Pestis in Two Forms

In the Introduction to Giovanni Boccaccio's *The Decameron* there is a fairly accurate description of the symptoms which accompany the Black Death. The year was 1348 in Italy; the plague had come from the East and was sweeping westward unhindered.

> . . . Toward the spring of the year the plague began to show its ravages in a way short of miraculous. It did not manifest itself as in the East, where if a man bled at the

... nose he had certain warning of inevitable death. At the onset of the disease both men and women were afflicted by a sort of swelling in the groin or under the armpits which sometimes attained the size of a common apple or egg. Some of these swellings were larger and some smaller, and all were commonly called boils. From these two starting points the boils began in a little while to spread and appear generally all over the body. Afterwards, the manifestation of the disease changed into black or livid spots on the arms, thighs and the whole person. In many, these blotches were large and far apart, in others small and closely clustered. Like the boils, which had been and continued to be a certain indication of coming death, these blotches had the same meaning for everyone on whom they appeared. . . .[2]

Again we find it mentioned that the disease occurred in different forms and with variable symptoms. The symptom of bleeding at the nose came from the form of pestis that affected the lungs, filling them with fluid and later with blood. About 25 percent of the cases were of this pneumonic type and were almost always fatal.

The other form of pestis had symptoms that appeared mainly as lymph node swellings in the groin and armpits. Other symptoms of this bubonic type were sudden high fever, headache, giddiness, sleeplessness, and pain in the back and limbs. Almost 75 percent of the cases of pestis in Europe were of the bubonic type, which was not always fatal. It is good to remember that if the bacteria invade the upper parts of the body, the lymph nodes of the armpits swell up, but if the lower parts of the body are invaded, the lymph nodes of the groin area become enlarged.

A rare form of pestis called septicemia, Greek for dirty blood, was an acute blood poisoning stemming from an invasion of the *Yersinia pestis* bacteria. This form of pestis was so severe that death ensued before either of the other two forms had time to appear, sometimes within twenty-four hours following infection.

These symptoms tell us that the pestis bacteria are extremely powerful, making the onset of disease rapid and severe in any of its forms. In humans, pestis is acute even in the milder bubonic cases where the latent period is only from two to ten days (compare this figure with tuberculosis, leprosy, or AIDS, where the time lapse may be a matter of years). These virulent characteristics put pestis in a class all of its own as an infectious and fatal disease. We are fortunate that AIDS takes a slower path.

Murakami's book on plagues mentions an author by the name of Lou Baker who wrote about the plague in England in 1349: " . . . the whole of England suffered heavily; only one in ten people survived. 'La Peste' attacked mainly young and strong people. The old, weak and sick escaped from illness and death."[3] This sounds very odd at first. It seems contrary to common sense, because we would expect old and weak people to be more susceptible to disease. A Japanese translation of the *Decameron* by Y. Nogami says, "The plague began from young men." Here young men means teenagers. An Arabian doctor named Al Razi (865-923) wrote, "Young people's blood is the same as fermenting wine, they are more vulnerable to the plague." Also, Agathias (536-582) wrote in his *The History of Byzantine*, "especially young active, vigorous men were afflicted more, less women had suffered." Did young people actually have the most favorable blood for the rapid growth of the pestis bacteria?

My answer is that in addition to flea bites, pestis was undoubtedly spread by intimate bodily contact, since it was bloodborne and highly contagious. Modern research has confirmed that bubonic pestis can be communicated by a droplet of fluid expelled by the infected person transmitted directly to a healthy subject. Boccaccio had observed that this could happen even in the course of visiting the sick. Also, two persons sharing the same bed and blankets would both be susceptible to the same fleas. The young and the strong became more rapidly infected by sharing fleas and sex, and Boccaccio also mentions that the youth ate a lot of meat and drank liquor. This lifestyle prepared their blood for the rapid onset of the disease and helped to spread the bacteria. Infectious disease develops from a combination of factors, being exposed to the pathogen and having the right conditions in the blood for the bacteria or virus to take hold and do its damage. Meat weakens the kidneys and alcohol damages the liver, causing a very poor blood quality in which bacteria can easily grow.

In the past, many historians have written that malnutrition from famine caused such disastrous plagues, but these reports are completely wrong. Seven to ten years prior to the plagues there were often famines or locust disasters, but I have never found famine and a pestilent plague occurring at the same time. Among all this suffering and death the physicians of those times were practically helpless. The only doctor who left marvellous records was Guy de Chauliac. He was originally a barber and belonged to that guild, but he had a special talent for medicine and his skill with the razor made him famous as the finest surgeon of Europe and the personal physician of Pope Clement VI. He wrote about pestis in his *Chirugia Magna,* dated 1363 (as translated in Murakami's book):

> I can definitely say this is the worst plague in history; past records show that such severity of affliction and death have never before occurred anywhere on Earth, with no exception. There has always been some kind of treatment for plagues, but this time nothing seems to work. . . . All physicians have hence become shameless and useless; they refuse to see patients for fear of catching the disease. Even if they do give an examination, they have nothing to prescribe and no treatment to perform. Besides, they cannot expect to be paid their medical fees, for all of their patients will eventually die. . . . I have only seen a few cases of people recovering; if the swelling buboes break open naturally and the pus is allowed to drain, they recovered.[4]

At the peak of the plague, the Pope sat down in his quarters and prayed to God. To repel the disease he made a fire in front of and behind himself and had a servant carry his food. This sounds like very strange protection, but fire can repel the rats and fleas, which were actually the cause of the plague. The Pope was safe. De Chauliac himself contracted the plague, and recovered in the way he describes. However, his most important contribution was his recommendations for preventing pestis:

> Do not eat poultry, the meat of young pigs, old cattle or any kind of fat-bearing animal. You can eat small fish from the river. Take soup cooked with a small amount of pepper, ginger, or clove. It is dangerous to use olive oil for cooking. It is good to drink wine a little bit at a time many times a day. Exposure to the sun is bad for fat people. Eat dinner one hour before sunset, retire early, and sleep well until the sun rises. Taking naps in the daytime is harmful; don't go out or stay out late at night.

It is amazing that de Chauliac wrote this over six hundred years ago. Animal meat, especially fatty meat, is dangerous because when it breaks down in the body it weakens the kidneys and makes the blood dirty and susceptible to bacterial growth. Pepper, ginger, and clove each have a strong medicinal power to neutralize the wastes built up from eating meat (they provide the vitamins and enzymes needed to break down the protein). He noted that people eating a lot of rich food tended to get pestis much more readily than thinner people who were on simpler, leaner diets. Olive oil was certainly used heavily, especially in Italy and France, and this is not beneficial for blood circulation. Wine was believed to have special properties of fortifying the blood and thus preventing disease; red wine is also high in iron (used for the blood's transport of oxygen) and a few sips throughout the day would help to counteract the effects of heavy meat-eating.

Spending too much time in the sun is bad especially for overweight people because it makes the blood more acid, which is conducive for the growth of bacteria. Since many people were overweight, de Chauliac emphasized this point many times.

Excessive acidity in the body causes the breathing to quicken and the heart to work harder, the body's automatic attempt to eliminate the acid. This situation is also especially dangerous for overweight people because their blood is usually thick and sticky as a result of the high-fat diet and their arteries are often very clogged. The recommendation to eat before sundown allows plenty of time for the food to be properly digested before going to bed. Eating and drinking at late night parties is not conducive to good health. During the great plague the wealthy urban people suffered more casualties than the poorer rural people. And finally, de Chauliac understood how promiscuity was conducive to the spread of pestis, so he recommended that people not go out at night when opportunities for sex would be more likely. Applying his opinion to the case of AIDS, we can see how accurate his perceptions are. This great physician could be considered one of the founders of preventive medicine. As you can see, we cannot find any trace of a starvation factor; every warning is directed to over-nourished people.

We can learn much more from the more modern scientific research of pestis. During 1893 and 1894 the southern part of China experienced a plague. Many researchers went to Hong Kong to try to find the causative microbe. A French doctor named Alexandre Yersin found the bacteria *Yersinia pestis*, and following this discovery certain kinds of rats were understood to be the bacteria carriers. Next fleas were discovered as the vector from the rats to the human body.

The relationship of rats and fleas having been established, the next question was whether or not the disease is contagious from human to human through the air. This was denied in medical research even though Boccaccio wrote, "the disease is transmitted by just visiting the patient." Later medical research discovered that the bacteria were found to be transmitted through the air from the droplets of patients. So, this is at the same time a bloodborne and an airborne diseae.

From these bitter experiences I want to say that it is too early to determine AIDS as a sexually transmitted disease. Reading reports from African research, the insect vector seems likely. One report says that AIDS is transmitted by the African bedbug, although about this airborne possibility I cannot say anything at this moment.

The research gets more exciting around 1910 when many Chinese moved into Manchuria. They hunted a special kind of rodent, sold the fur at very good prices, ate the meat, and started pestis. The Mongolian people who lived in this area had a taboo against hunting or eating this animal, especially strongly prohibiting the eating of the lymph nodes of the animal.

The disease spread to China and devastated its southern territories. From Hong Kong the bacteria rode on trading boats and spread all over the world. Thus it was called the Hong Kong plague. An estimated 100 million people died, but compared to the entire world population, this number was not extremely large. The most frightening fact is that the disease started from eating the meat of infected animals. Although we don't know where the AIDS virus originated in humans, it is not impossible to think that people ate the meat of green monkeys and got the disease, if the green monkey is considered to be the original virus carrier.

Diet and the Different Forms of Disease

Now we can review what we have learned from these epidemics and plagues to see how it pertains to our present-day problem with AIDS and to the prevention of any other potentially epidemic catastrophes. In each of the examples given – leprosy, tuberculosis, and pestis, along with the previous discussion about AIDS – two distinct forms of each disease appear, even though only one kind of bacteria or virus is associated as the pathogen. In the previous chapter the concept of balance between two types of foods also was introduced. This concept is repeated here with further explanation.

Our food can be classified easily into two categories: animal and animal-derived, and plant and plant-derived. (A third category is that of minerals, including water and salt, substances that are not usually considered to be foods, even though they, like the air we breathe, should be.) When we eat too much animal food, usually in the form of meat, our body becomes susceptible to a pyogenic (pus producing) form of infection, a destructive type of disease. Such a disease usually appears on the skin (as a result of malfunctioning kidneys) and in the lower part of the body, generally on the surface. This type of disease can affect strong people and can come and go more quickly. Kaposi's sarcoma, typical leprosy, the warty form of tuberculosis, and the bubonic form of pestis are all examples of destructive diseases.

As we saw during the time of the Great Plague, people from Eastern countries died mainly from pneumonic pestis; at that time they already were consuming honey and sugar. When we eat too much of certain plant-derived foods, usually in refined forms such as sugar, we become more susceptible to a degenerative type of disease. These attack the lungs, the brain, and the nervous system mainly in the upper parts of the body first and are generally more internalized and not so apparent on the surface as the destructive type. *Pneumocystosis carinii* pneumonia, tuberculoid leprosy, typical tuberculosis, and pneumonic pestis are examples of the diseases associated with eating sweeteners and/or drinking a lot of alcohol. They are generally the slow-acting and slow-to-heal diseases of weaker people. These I call the degenerative diseases.

A third type of disease results from habitual excesses of both categories of food, for example, meat and sugar. If both are taken in small amounts, our bodies are capable of neutralizing them. But if both are consumed in excess, then the bad effects of each accumulate, leading to a clearly destructive outcome such as a septicemic disease.

Actually, diseases are more complicated. But if you understand the two typical forms, variations are easier to comprehend as combinations of these two basic types. The concept of two types of food in relation to disease will be repeated and developed throughout this book. I would like to clarify that I am referring to habitual patterns of diet, not just a meal or two. These dietary patterns eventually build up toxic excesses that weaken various organs, lead to their degeneration or destruction, and place undue strain on other organs and systems. We will now see how excessive meat-eating is destructive to the body.

Chapter 3

The Meat-Eater's Body

Strong Bodies are More Susceptible

Chapter Two introduced the ancient observation that the plague attacked the young and the strong. It seems to go against common sense, but this is correct.

Our image of a strong body is usually one with hard muscles suitable for fighting or heavy physical work. Before our ancestors developed weapons, men of this type could win battles against large predators like lions or wolves. They became leaders among their peers since fighting was long necessary for survival. With heavy meat-eating and hard training, they were also able to dominate other men. Many wanted to be in this position and have this kind of body. Later, when populations had increased, the physically strong were able to manipulate people and weapons with skill, thus becoming lords or kings. Nevertheless, these great heroes were often vulnerable to disease.

One of the most famous men in the Western world was Alexander the Great, who died of a high fever infection at the age of thirty-three. In China the first Great Emperor, Shih Huang Ti, who built the Great Wall and of whom it is said that he had three thousand mistresses in his harem, died at the age of forty-eight of an acute infection. In more recent times records are more clear.

45

Henry VIII (1491-1547) had a big body, was an excellent athlete, and was a tireless hunter and dancer. After he became king, much animal food was consumed during the continuous feasts both day and night. He married six times and frequently visited prostitutes. It is said that during his reign 3 percent of London's population, including two of his wives and his prime minister, Sir Thomas Moore, were killed. In his thirties he had gout. When he died at the age of fifty-five, he had kidney disease, gout, circulatory disease, syphilis, and ulcers. In King Henry's case, many people agree that his real trouble was food.

Throughout history the strong man has been admired and men have tried to grow stronger and stronger. In modern society such a body type is not so useful, but many young girls still admire such bodies. Many young men, through body-building techniques and high-protein diets, try to produce a strong, muscular body. This kind of body is weak, especially for superlative or purulent forms of infections and high fevers. So, this is a dangerous fad. I do not recommend such foods and training. In a healthy body our muscles should be soft when we relax and become hard when we use them.

In the last one hundred years, with the development of microscopic research, we have discovered that microorganisms invade the human body and cause infections. These microbes we call the causative agents, or pathogens, of disease. A so-called strong body against large predators is clearly weaker against microorganisms. We have to change the image to one where strong means never defeated by microbes.

One Man Eats Twenty-five Cattle

Americans now eat about 250 pounds of meat per person per year on the average. In the past three hundred years meat consumption has increased significantly, especially in the last one hundred years. For instance, in 1850 meat consumption in the United States was estimated at seventy-five pounds per person per year. If we calculate the weight of one cow as one thousand pounds with an edible part of about seven hundred pounds, then during seventy years of life, one person eats about twenty-five cows. It is hard to believe that to maintain two hundred pounds of body weight for seventy years, one eats 17,500 pounds of meat. In contrast, today in Lebanon annual consumption per person is only twelve pounds, so we can see that Americans were eating six times as much meat in 1850 as the Lebanese are now.

Large Body, Early Maturity

The American people are the pioneers of a new diet – the milk, meat, and sugar diet – and a large body has been one result. We can see what has happened in the last hundred years: From birth, babies are fed with cow's milk, which is richer in protein than mother's milk but not as sweet; sugar is then added, so the babies grow quickly and learn the taste of sugar. Later, every child develops a sweet tooth, as well as a desire for high protein foods such as eggs and meat. This is natural for balancing their nutrition. When they are fifteen years old, the children are often as big as their parents.

Around this age teenage problems often begin, clearly showing an imbalance of physical and mental development. Physically they have matured, but there is no way to artificially speed up mental development. Statistics show that as many as 27 percent of teenagers misuse alcohol and that the crime rate also is increasing. They seem to have no self-control. In the last hundred years menstruation in American girls has begun two and one-half years earlier – from fifteen and one-half to thirteen years of age.[1] It is not unusual to find fifteen-year-old mothers. If the babies are healthy this is not bad because a large population is the power of a nation. But often the babies are weak and the fathers of such babies have no ability to support the family's living expenses, and government help may be necessary. An estimated one million babies are born each year from teenage mothers in the United States.

So we have succeeded in building larger bodies, but this acquired character needs hundreds of generations for genetic assimilation before a big body becomes hereditary. Such a body is not suitable for the world, for, unfortunately, this kind of body is not strong against infections. It is possible for humans to disappear from this world.

This is clear evidence. For the past hundred years Americans have been building up this kind of meat-eater's body, which has been the most important co-factor in weakening the immune system and causing the development of AIDS. But it is not by chance that very few women have developed AIDS, especially in the United States. I believe that American men consume more than twice as much meat as do women. This is why AIDS is a disease that primarily affects males in this country. On the average, a woman's lifespan is longer. A woman's muscles are generally softer than a man's and so she has more resistance to infections and many other kinds of diseases except those related to the female organs. Also, the fact that men eat more meat than women is worldwide. Probably this dates back to the Stone Age, when men did the hunting and ate more meat, while women remained at home to care for the children. They gathered and ate more grains, nuts, and seeds. If men want to live long and healthy lives, it may be good to learn from women.

In Africa an almost equal number of men and women have contracted AIDS (the ratio is 10:9), but the incidences of Kaposi's sarcoma are eight times greater among men.[2] This is because KS is a disease mainly caused by excess consumption of meat. As African women are for the most part vegetarians, they do not fall prey to this type of tumor. Sugar, as we will see in the next chapter, influences the direction of AIDS or other diseases where KS does not develop.

Sex-related Problems

From the many doctors' reports I have read of interviews with AIDS patients, I have learned that these patients had far more active sexual lives than average. One man is reported to have had sex twenty-five times in one week and another had more than a thousand sex partners in one year.[3] This number exceeds within one year the whole-life record of the famous Don Juan and is more than ten times the average of American sexual practices, according to Dr. Kinsey's reports.

About one case the interviewing doctor writes: "He lives for sex – the more unusual 'kinky' sex he can find, the better. He's obsessed by sex, addicted to it, and he has arranged his entire life so that nothing else will interfere with his pursuit of sex."[4] While this case is not necessarily typical, it does point out the relevance of excessive sexual activity as a co-factor in the development of AIDS.

However, I understand why so many men want to eat large quantities of meat, and why women support this desire of meat-eating. Men lose a lot of the body's protein during sex, as the semen and seminal fluid are largely protein, and this depletion creates an appetite for more meat, which in turn increases the sex drive, which depletes the body, which creates a hunger for meat, and so on. Sex and morality are not my subjects of discussion here; every person's sexual life is private. My interest is only in health and long life. If you are healthy and happy you can do as you wish, but if you eat meat to stimulate sex, I feel this is dangerous to your health.

The Main Nutrition

The major nutrients of our bodies can be viewed as fuel material and building material. Fuel material, also called the energy source, can be classified further as carbohydrates and fat, the primary sources of producing heat to keep the body warm and of maintaining the functions of the organs and muscles. A large amount of fuel material is consumed by the body and needs to be constantly supplied from food.

Protein, the most plentiful substance in the body, is the major source of building material for muscle, blood, skin, hair, nails, and the internal organs. It is needed for the formation of hormones and blood coagulants, as well as to replace parts of the body that are constantly being lost or destroyed through metabolism and excretion. One very important thing to understand is that under normal circumstances it is not necessary to take large amounts of protein.

Our bodies cannot store large amounts of protein. There is no way to excrete excess protein, which the body must break down into carbohydrates for use as fuel even before it uses existing supplies of other carbohydrates and fat. Biologically this is the most economical way for the body to utilize its nutrition.

It appears that protein is the most useful nutrient since it can be used for building material and fuel material. Carbohydrates and fat are only used as materials for fuel and not as building materials. If we have a protein shortage in the body, this is considered malnutrition despite an excess of carbohydrates and fat. This is reasonable, but a big mistake has been made. The useful side of protein has been well understood, but the harmful side of the effects of excess protein has not.

The Harmful Effects of Meat-Eating

The first danger of eating meat is that the protein level of the blood goes up temporarily. This creates a more dangerous condition for infection. The main nutrition of microbes is also protein. Excess protein provides good nutrition for the microbes to increase. The increased acid in the blood from the breakdown of the protein makes a better environment for microbes. Many kinds of germs which cause disease, especially many kinds of fungi, favor and are strong in a slightly acid condition which is toxic for our body cells.

The second problem with meat eating is that it overloads the liver and kidneys. Protein is different from carbohydrates and fat in that protein contains nitrogen in addition to carbon, hydrogen, and oxygen. When the protein is broken down by the liver, our chemical factory, the nitrogen is removed in the making of ammonia. But this ammonia is quite toxic for the body cells, so it is immediately converted to urea. Animal meat contains large amounts of protein, fat, and a crystalline compound which produces a group of compounds known as purines. Uric acid is produced by the breakdown of purines. Also sulfur and phosphorous in the meat turn into sulfuric and phosphoric acid in the body. All these kinds of side-products are sent into the bloodstream. The kidneys receive and filtrate this blood, reabsorbing useful materials and excreting useless or harmful substances. If the kidneys can not filtrate all the wastes, the body has trouble from the excess.

Another problem is that meat does not contain enough minerals, vitamins, or dietary fiber. Human nutrition requires more than the three major nutrients; many kinds of minerals and vitamins are also needed. Some minerals and vitamins are high enough in meat but others are missing. Dietary fiber is not required nutritionally but it has an important function in the elimination of wastes from the body. Meat does not contain this material. Plant foods are a better form of nutrition and contain more varieties of nutrients and fiber.

Moreover, meat often contains microbes which cause disease in humans. More about this later.

What is really needed by the body are the building blocks of protein, the amino acids. All the sources of protein that we eat are first broken down into the component amino acids so that our body can reassemble them into the various proteins it needs. The amino acids we need are most complete and balanced in mammal's meat and this is why it has been so widely accepted as the best source. Surely, animal meat seems like the shortest and easiest way to obtain protein, but this is a poor quality of protein. Our body can easily compose perfect amino acids from a combination of plant foods. Protein derived from vegetal sources is considered the best, for this protein is brand new. If you eat meat, your body is recycling used protein at a high cost. Dirty materials result from this recycling process; besides the amino acids obtained when these animal proteins are broken down, there are many toxic waste products that must be excreted. For this reason, eating meat all the time is not a good practice.

Meat Warms the Body

We know that meat is a concentrated high-protein food that also contains fat, cholesterol, and sodium, but what happens to it inside the body?

You may have experienced how eating meat warms the body, increases thirst, and stops the urge to urinate. When you do urinate, it is dark and thick and has a strong odor. The principle of homeostasis, the regulation of the body, has been at work. Specifically, the amount of protein in the body has increased, causing a temporary imbalance with the other components of the blood. The body then craves water for diluting thick blood, and sugar in some form – an alcoholic drink, for example – in order to compensate for the protein overload. The excess protein then overstimulates the nervous and endocrine systems. This stimulation typically results in restless sleep, a strong desire for sex, bed sweating at times, a higher body temperature, a quickening of the pulse, ringing in the ears, and other effects.

Eating meat does make the body warmer, so it is a suitable food in winter and in the polar zones where the weather is always cold. In cold weather the side-effects of eating meat are not so strong. Eskimos eat a diet of about 90 percent raw meat with a small amount of sea vegetables. Crops such as grains, vegetables, and fruits don't grow in those climates, yet people stay healthy without them. Physical activity also eliminates the undesirable effects of eating meat; active cell metabolism uses more protein and allows many of the waste products to be excreted through the skin in the form of sweat.

In the United States the climate is generally temperate and the native products are chiefly grains, beans, vegetables, seeds, and some fruits and nuts; our diet should consist primarily of these foods with small amounts of meat or animal foods from time to time.

Why does meat-eating make our bodies warmer? Everyone knows that meat and especially poultry makes the body warmer; so, many people eat more chicken in the wintertime. If it were just a question of calories, one gram of fat produces nine kilocalories while one gram of protein or carbohydrate each make four kilocalories. But the question is more than this because some nuts and seeds contain more fat than chicken, yet if we eat nuts and seeds, we don't feel as warm as when we eat chicken.

Calorie research has been done by burning each nutrient, but this is a rather primitive method. Rudolf Steiner proposed a new research method using the sun's energy, but this is difficult to measure. Another method was tested by keeping a man in a closed room and feeding him certain kinds of food and measuring how many calories his body produced and lost, but still the answer is not clear.

Probably there are quick-burning foods and slow-burning foods. Animal meat, especially chicken, is a quick-burning food, like high octane fuel. Plant foods burn more slowly but last for a longer time. Another idea is that the process of nitrogen separating from protein produces heat, for when plants synthesize protein they absorb more sunshine than carbohydrates or fat. Much more research is needed.

Unbalanced Minerals

The problem with meat is not only with the main nutrients but also with minerals. Meat does not have enough minerals except for phosphorous, potassium, and sulphur. Meats contain some calcium, but the amounts are rather low; sodium is not so low. Chlorine, magnesium, and many other trace elements are absolutely in short supply. Some vitamins like thiamine, niacin, and ascorbic acid are insufficient.

After meat is eaten, it is considered good practice to take more tea, coffee, or other liquid because the body needs to dilute the high concentration of protein; consequently, the mineral and vitamin contents decrease relatively speaking. To cover this nutrition shortage, it is good to eat vegetables, since vegetables also contain the best quality of water. But these are bulky, so many people take supplements instead. What is missing here is dietary fiber.

In the intestines, meat causes fermentation to occur and produces indole, skatole, methane, and other gases.[5] These toxic gases dissolve in the water and enter the bloodstream through the intestinal wall. These undesirables along with uric acid and other acids combine and make the dirty blood which the ancient Greeks called septicemia. The kidneys are mainly responsible for cleansing the blood of these waste products, working without a moment's rest, twenty-four hours a day, every day.[6] Eating vegetables helps ease the load on the kidneys because vegetables can neutralize a lot of the acid. Many people now consume amounts of meat beyond the cleansing capabilities of the kidneys; this is fatal for many of the body cells, including white blood cells. Septicemia is one trouble which disappeared after the practical use of antibiotics. This was once a prevalent and dreaded infection; patients often died within two days of the onset of the disease. They had immune deficiency symptoms, but before the etiology was clarified the trouble had diminished.

Skin Helps the Kidneys

When too much meat is ingested, the blood becomes excessively acid and the kidneys become overloaded. The waste materials not cleaned by the kidneys have to get out of the body somehow. For the vitality and stability of the body cells, homeostasis must be achieved. The backup for the kidneys is the skin, the main contact with the external environment and the largest organ of the body. The skin has been called the third kidney because of its eliminative functions in cleansing acids in the blood, toxins, and mineral wastes.[7] These materials exit through the skin with the sweat, often causing a strong body odor. Excess dirt from these wastes is also brought to the surface of the skin, requiring the use of strong soaps in a hot bath or shower. Many chemically harsh soaps, deodorants, shampoos, and skin cleansers were developed to deal with the conditions mainly caused by increased meat consumption. For vegetarians this is not only needless but also a harmful practice. If we wash away all the skin's excretions, we also lose some important materials such as sebum and salt. Sebum is the oil which the sebaceous glands excrete to protect the skin and help keep it smooth, flexible, and shiny. It also contains an untimicrobial substance. To clean the skin, washing with plain water is good enough; rub your skin with a towel or brush.

We cannot see the inner organs but we can see by the skin if something has changed. The skin is the clearest signal of the onset of many diseases, as we saw in the first chapter. To neglect the signs your skin gives you is like ignoring traffic signals; both can be essential for your life. Changes in the appearance of your skin can tell you that you have had enough meat and should stop for awhile. If not, infection may soon set in.

Skin Diseases

With continued meat-eating, the skin produces scurf, dandruff, and scales; then pimples, acne, and finally skin rashes. These problems are worsened by bacteria, fungi, and dirt. The condition can be further aggravated as more serious diseases and infections develop, such as skin ulcers, eczema, and psoriasis. The body is trying to throw out all toxic wastes as quickly as possible. The kidneys can only do so much of the work; when they are overloaded it is up to the skin to keep the blood clean. Treating a skin disease with strong medications can cure it, but this often leads to kidney disease which is much more difficult to cure and can sometimes be disastrous. A symptomatic treatment without an understanding of how the condition came about will only lead to further complications and ill health.

There are hundreds of different kinds of skin diseases, but the cause is always the same – the kidneys cannot handle all the wastes produced by the food we eat. Many different food combinations, along with the types of bacteria or fungi present, account for these varieties.

Digestion and Constipation

The mouth is connected to the anus by the digestive tube, some thirty feet long. Things have to be kept moving in this tube or they will ferment and putrify. This movement is essential for our blood quality and good health. If you were to take a typical American meal of meat and sugar, mix it all together, add some intestinal bacteria, and incubate it at about 100°F for a couple of days, you would get an idea of what happens inside the body after eating such a meal. It turns rotten and smells very bad. We can compare the feces of cats and horses. Cats know the smell is bad, so they cover them with sand or dirt; horses are vegetarian and their feces smell a little like green tea and they never cover them with dirt.

The presence of dietary fiber in the colon stimulates the intestinal walls to move constantly. Sugar and meat contain no fiber and have very few indigestible substances to provide the necessary bulk for the intestinal muscles to work against. The result of this lack of stimulation is constipation; dense and fiberless food can stay in the colon for days at a time. This longer retention means more water is absorbed, leaving the feces dry, hard, and difficult to evacuate.

Normally the colon produces mucus to protect the intestinal wall and to keep the movement of material constant, smooth, and continuous. But once constipation sets in, the colon loses its mucus when the water is absorbed, and the feces attach themselves directly to the intestinal wall. Even small amounts of this material on the walls of the colon can accumulate over a long period of time to form a toxic coat that is responsible for many chronic diseases. Constipation causes many discomforts, including loss of appetite, headaches, acne, hemorrhoids, and varicose veins, and is usually the first step in colon diseases such as colitis, appendicitis, diverticulitis, and colon cancer. It is well known that many heart attacks occur in the morning, but most people don't know why. If you have a normal elimination in the morning, a heart attack can be avoided.

In the United States alone, we spend about half a billion dollars per year on laxatives, but they cannot resolve this problem. Soon they become habit-forming and we need larger doses. Some laxatives cause malabsorption of nutrients, leading to chronic conditions such as osteomalacia. Wheat bran is better than other laxatives; it is more natural and has no side-effects, but it is best to take whole wheat bread instead of separated bran. Also, it is better to reduce the meat intake and increase the fresh vegetables.

All foods should be taken in as natural a form as possible, the way nature provides us. Food supplements of any kind should be taken only on special occasions for specific conditions or problems.

Foods like whole grains and especially beans are high in fiber, providing the indigestible bulk which allows a constant movement of the feces through and out of the body. If you are eating meat and thereby creating toxic acids, however, vegetables are better – they neutralize the acids and also provide the necessary fiber to prevent constipation. Raw vegetables are more undigestible and have more vitamin C than cooked vegetables, so they are well suited for meat-eaters.

Effects of Different Animal Foods

Now we can see that meat has both a strong constructive effect (+) and a strong destructive effect (-) on the body. Further, there are many different kinds of meat and each has a slightly different effect than the other. Generally, dark red meat such as beef, lamb, venison, and other meat of mammals (the most like human flesh) are the strongest. We can show the comparison with these symbols: Red meat (++++); poultry and eggs (+++); then fish (++); the white meat of shrimp, crab, octopus, and many other kinds of shellfish (+). Dairy products, such as milk, cheese, and yogurt are almost neutral in that they are between animal food and plant food. At one time they were good foods, but now the quality of milk has changed. This is discussed in a later chapter.

Henry Bieler, M.D., suggests that the best way to eat meat is raw.[8] It is easier to digest and less toxic effects have been noted.

This is true if the meat is not contaminated by causative germs of diseases. But, surprising evidence of the danger of meat-eating comes from the work of Dr. Roderick, quoted in Dr. Hoffman's book on the Hunzas.[9]

> Dr. C. E. Roderick, bacteriologist of the laboratory of the Battle Creek Sanitarium, recently made, at the request of the writer, an extended study of the bacteria of meat and of the fresh droppings of animals. Specimens of meat were purchased from seven different markets. The bacteria found were identical with those found in fresh manure and in several instances the bacteria in meat exceeded in number those of fresh manure.
>
> Meats – Bacteria per gram
>
> | | |
> |---|---:|
> | Beefsteak | 1,500,000 |
> | Corned beef | 31,000,000 |
> | Hamburger steak | 75,000,000 |
> | Pork liver | 95,000,000 |
> | Limburger cheese | 18,000,000 |
> | Oyster juice | 3,400,000 |
>
> Droppings of Animals – Bacteria per gram
>
> | | |
> |---|---:|
> | Fresh droppings of calf | 15,000,000 |
> | Fresh droppings of goat | 20,000,000 |
> | Fresh droppings of horse | 25,000,000 |

It is evident that any flesh that is eaten is to some degree unsafe. Ordinary cooking does not destroy the germs in meat. They are killed only by a temperature of 240°F and the oven heat does not penetrate to the interior of the roast. This means it is possible to get diseases caused by eating meat, whether raw or cooked.

Food Reactions

Some people may experience strong reactions if they suddenly stop eating meat entirely. Many of these reactions are especially well-known to people who have fasted as a means of cleansing the body. The natural regenerative and cleansing action of the body works to push out accumulated toxins and needless materials and waste, and this process can cause headaches, nausea, body odors, bed sweating, and some body aches and pains. These are signs that better health is on the way, so there is no need to worry. These symptoms will go away within several days. You may notice a redness in your extremities as bad blood is released into the system to be eliminated, or a thick coating of white or yellow material on your tongue, especially in the morning. If you also stop eating dairy products, you can expect a runny nose and some coughing up of phlegm as the built-up mucus is being discharged from the internal tissues.

Special Advice for Pregnant Women

A sudden change in diet is not recommended for pregnant women and nursing mothers. During pregnancy this can initiate the process of discharge and force many of the toxic wastes into the fetus. A weak baby may result. But if you have been vegetarian for more than three years, you won't have this problem. For pregnant women and nursing mothers who have been meat-eaters, I suggest a weekly ration of either a quarter pound of meat (preferably chicken or turkey) or one to two or three eggs or half a pound of fish. This is for each week until the baby is old enough to begin eating some solid foods (usually at about six months).

After Four Months Vegetarian

As an AIDS prevention practice I recommend a four-month blood cleansing period using a grain and vegetable diet. This came from my own experiments and observations, but modern hematology also affirms that our red blood cells survive in the circulatory system for about 120 days. This means that within four months our blood has been completely renewed. If after this four-month period you are not overweight and your muscles are not hard, you may follow a lacto-ovo-vegetarian diet (eggs and dairy products allowed). Watch for the hidden contents of processed foods; it's surprising how many breads and other foods contain eggs. One egg a day should be maximum, or one pound of meat per week – that means you can eat two or three ounces of meat per day, or a quarter of a pound four times a week. This is not a recommendation, but one suggestion for a way to begin dietary change.

Even with this reduced amount of meat, you may still consume more than five cattle in your seventy years of life. With that amount you will never have a protein deficiency. But if you contract AIDS, you will not be able to eat even one animal meal in the next two years.

There is one more very important item in the typical everyday diet that is a serious threat to health: sugar. The next chapter will look at this primary degenerative factor in the development of disease.

Chapter 4

Sugar

Highly Processed Food

In order to evolve, our primitive ancestors developed the ability to judge the value of many kinds of foods and tastes. The need for salt developed at the early stage of ocean life and now the entire tongue can taste salt. Then it was necessary to recognize bitter foods which may contain fatal poisons; this is sensed at the back of the tongue. Next, the sour or acid taste was developed, as wild plants which contain the acid taste were added to the diet, and this is felt at the sides of the tongue. Finally, our ancestors began eating grains, tubers (potatoes), and fruits and they acquired the sweet taste, located at the front of the tongue. These sugars assisted brain development, which coincided with stronger lungs for oxygen intake and the more upright posture.

Many kinds of naturally growing foods contain nutrients our bodies need. But humans liked the sweet taste and our ancestors always looked for sweeter food. They discovered honey and also developed fermentation and syrup concentrates.

Five hundred years ago, not many people knew about sugar. At that time, sugar was still in an unrefined form. Now if we say sugar we mean the pure white or colored, completely refined table variety. To cultivate, extract, and refine sugar highly developed techniques are needed; so, at one time sugar was thought of as the most developed food.

However, from the viewpoint of complete nutrition, sugar is the most degraded food, providing the possibility of leading us to a degraded body and inviting degenerative diseases. From this point of view, honey and other syrups are a little better because they contain some other nutrients, but still the sugar content is very high and they are very sweet.

At one time in history, sugar was considered a medicine that only the rich could afford. Most sugar is a product of tropical areas, so it is usually an imported food in this country. The price of sugar is now so low that it is available almost everywhere.

Statistics now indicate that sugar consumption for Americans is about 140 pounds per person per year, including corn syrup, maple syrup, honey, and beet sugar.[1] The only other foods Americans eat more of are red meat and wheat flour. It is likely that the availability and popularity of sugar is what made the huge increase in meat consumption possible. This chapter will explain the connection between these two kinds of foods. It will also touch upon what sugar is, why people eat so much of it, what effects it has on the body, and how it contributes to a wide variety of diseases, including AIDS.

Is Sweetness Necessary?

The sugars and starches found in grains, potatoes, fruits, honey, corn syrup, table sugar, etc., all belong to the class of foods called carbohydrates, the main components of which are carbon, oxygen, and hydrogen. Alcohol, also made from carbohydrates, has a similar chemical structure and a similar effect as sugar. Carbohydrates are the chief source of energy for all bodily functions and muscular exertion. They also help to regulate protein and fat metabolism, and are necessary for the digestion and assimilation of other nutrients. Sweet or not, carbohydrates of various types from numerous sources are converted by the saliva and digestive juices into a simple sugar or monosaccharide. This enters the bloodstream as glucose, commonly called blood sugar, and provides the calories or energy we need to produce heat in the body. The brain tissues are the biggest consumers of blood sugar, followed by the muscles and the nervous system. If enough energy is supplied, it is not necessary for the food to be sweet; for example, lactose (mother's milk) is not so sweet – only about one-sixth as sweet as table sugar.

In order for the modern, developed human brain to maintain and support its activity, glucose (taken from our food) and oxygen (from the air) are essential. Research studies in physiology indicate that the brain consumes about 20 percent of the glucose in the blood and more than 25 percent of the oxygen taken in by the lungs. These are the amounts for ordinary maintenance and activity when the brain is at rest. When we use our brain for thinking, concentrating, or other mental work, oxygen consumption increases to about 33 percent; many researchers say the glucose consumption does not change very much. But once the blood sugar goes down, as in hypoglycemia, the brain does not work well, suggesting the strong relationship between the brain and sugar. PET scanner examinations also show that the active brain cell consumes more glucose.[2]

In our age, machines have largely replaced human physical labor and the majority of the population is engaged in mental work. It is reasonable to eat more sugar for this mental activity, but it has now become excessive. As mentioned, the average American consumes about 140 pounds of sugar per year. That is almost the same as the average body weight. In one life span of seventy years, one person eats about five tons of sugar. Much research is being done on disorders such as diabetes and obesity.[3] Thus, the public is becoming more aware of the connection between these illnesses and the intake of sugar, and this is only the beginning.

Sugar and Alcohol
Sugar turns into alcohol by the process of fermentation, usually

derived from the carbohydrates of plants. Although the chemical formulas of alcohol and sugar are similar and they have similar effects, sugar is worse than alcohol, in my opinion, because its effects are not as well understood. Sugar degenerates the body without our awareness, while alcohol is honest: the skin color changes, the breath smells strong, and emotions surface. But within twenty-four hours the alcohol disappears from the body. Excess consumption can cause liver trouble, brain damage, and other diseases, but small amounts can be enjoyed from time to time if you are not prone to car accidents, fights, or strong emotions when you take alcoholic drinks.

Traditionally, alcohol was thought of as a man's food, while fruit and sugar were favored by women and children. Before refined sugar consumption became widespread, our cravings for the sweet taste were satisfied by fruit, certainly a far better source. Men had their meat and alcohol and women and children had sweets. This pattern still persists all over the world. When I saw the United States statistics for the first time, I was surprised to learn that men were consuming more sugar than women. But when I looked carefully at the situation, I saw that teenage boys were the biggest consumers of sugar. However, after the age of puberty their interest goes to sex rather than sugar; this is quite normal and would account for these statistics.

Sugar and Meat Balance

We know that the per capita consumption of meat in this country increased about 30 percent between 1901 and 1975. In the same period, sugar consumption doubled (100 percent) and the intake of ice cream increased five hundred times. We have seen how meat can be harmful to health by weakening the immune system, but were it not for sugar, people would not eat so much meat. This is a very important cycle to understand: sugar drives you to eat meat, while excessive meat intake creates a craving for sugar, and so on.

The all-important function and maintenance of homeostasis

requires that the condition of the blood and its various components along with the body fluids be kept constant and stable. Almost all our organs – the brain and the nervous and endocrine systems – must work together to perform this formidable task. From a biological point of view, our trillions of individual cells are the citizens of the body; their protective or adaptive mechanisms are the totality of the body's millions of years of experience and intelligence. The different conditions in our external environment – heat and cold, danger and safety, sexual stimulation, etc. – and the substances we ingest that form the internal environment, such as air, water, and food, all bring this elaborate and wonderful biological system, the body, into action.

As we found in the last chapter, meat-eating increases the proportion of various amino and fatty acids in the blood, along with the levels of sodium, phosphorus, sulfur, and other substances. Immediately the body begins to reestablish homeostasis by adjusting these levels. First, certain cravings appear. We want to drink water, coffee, tea, alcohol, or other liquids to dilute the proteins, fats, acids, and other substances. The next urgent task is to adjust the glucose (blood sugar) content; the body wants fruits, cakes, ice cream, or other desserts. The healthiest way to adjust this imbalance is to eat vegetables, but this means large amounts of salad or cooked vegetables. Fruits are higher in sugar so less volume is needed to restore balance. Fruit sugar (fructose) enters the intestine quickly and turns to glucose. Grains and other complex carbohydrates also change to glucose, but many hours are needed to digest these foods, so they are not as effective for an urgent need.

Body-Cooling Food

Sugars and proteins always work together, although the effect of each is opposite. Meat creates warmth in the body in combination with sugar, but an excess of sugar will outbalance the protein and make the body cold. Sugar alone never burns without protein and other minerals and vitamins. The production of body heat is a great symphony of many kinds of nutrients and enzymes. Excess sugar makes the body tired and lacking in energy, creating a craving for meat, and the meat-sugar cycle can begin again. Many people play this seesaw game every day. Sugar also cools down sexual desire and reduces sexual ability, and leads to frigidity, impotency, and sterility. The reasons will be discussed later, but for now just remember that it has the opposite effect of meat.

However, the undesirable effects of sugar go far beyond its interaction with meat. When I say sugar, I am speaking of all natural sweets which contain sugar of various forms: cane and beet sugar, honey, corn syrup, maple syrup, and sometimes in the wider meaning it includes fruit and other foods with an extremely sweet taste. The purest refined white sugar processed from cane or sugar beets, sucrose, contains no protein, no minerals, no vitamins, and no fiber. It is more than 99 percent pure simple carbohydrate, more like a chemical drug. When it enters the body, it quickly turns to glucose, the blood sugar. This is needless haste; the body never needs such quick energy. Despite research findings that have been reported about the dangers of quickly elevated sugar levels in the blood, especially on a daily basis, people continue to consume sugar pound after pound. Furthermore, excess sugar does not burn well in the body; its combustion is similar to a smoky fire.

The Nutrient Thief

Sugar's worst effect is that it robs us of essential nutrients. It removes calcium and other minerals, depletes our stores of protein, and consumes important nutrients like vitamin B_1.

Calcium is the major building material of bones and teeth. The skeleton holds about 98 percent of the body's calcium, while the teeth have about 1 percent. The remaining 1 percent is used through the body for the regulation of muscle function (especially the heart), the clotting of blood, nourishment of cells, release of energy, and transmission of nerve impulses; in the stomach, calcium restrains excessive acid secretion and neutralizes various detrimental food additives. The calcium ion protects our body from the virulent character of the sodium and potassium ions, copper, and other metals, and also helps to regulate body temperature. For all these reasons calcium is one of the most important minerals.

Since calcium loss is difficult to test on humans, the only thing I can do is to illustrate with examples. If you are interested in laboratory tests conducted on animals, please read Dr. J. Yudkin's book, *Sweet and Dangerous*.[4]

On this point – that sugar removes calcium – scientists do not agree. It seems they are saying that nothing has been proven, so I have to make this clear. The fact that sugar requires a person to take more water in some form to dilute it cannot be neglected by anyone. If a person eats cake or candy, that person will want to drink tea, coffee, plain water, or something. If one doesn't eat sweets, then the excess liquid intake is not wanted. Normally, one or two cups of black coffee are enough for anyone to be satisfied, but if sugar is added, the taste is too good and thus some people drink much more. If soft drinks were not sweet, not many people would drink them. These are all examples of excess liquid, beyond our biological necessity.

Is Water or Sugar to Blame?

For the average person, drinking water is calculated to be four to five cups per day. More water is consumed as a component of food. Urination is about five to six cups per person per day. But many Americans are drinking much more in many forms. Beer consumption is about six billion gallons per year, or an average of twenty-five gallons per person per year. Coffee and soft drink consumption are higher than beer. However, milk is consumed in the largest amount. Milk is actually a food, but because of the high water content, it is also a kind of beverage. As a total, some people are drinking more than one gallon per day in excess.

As a result, some people are urinating more than ten cups a day. Human urine contains about 0.015 percent of calcium. In five cups of urine, one excretes about 0.075 grams per day. If one drinks excess liquid and urinates five additional cups of urine, this makes 0.15 grams per day. In fifty years time, the calcium loss is totalled to be about 13.5 kilograms or about three pounds for five cups of urine per day and about 27 kilograms or about six pounds for ten cups per day. The adult body has an average of about three pounds of calcium and three pounds of calcium loss is considered normal. This much calcium is replaced from daily food intake. However, if the body loses six pounds of calcium, this is harder to replace. Drinking milk or taking calcium pills will not compensate for this huge loss.

This is just one example. In the same way, many other minerals, vitamins, and even hormones are lost from excess urination caused by excess liquid intake which in turn is caused by eating excess amounts of sugar.

Dental Caries

There is a strong correlation between sugar consumption and the prevalence of caries or decayed teeth because of the calcium loss. The reason given is that the bacterial fermentation in the mouth produces organic acids which make the teeth decay, but this does not seem right. Despite the popularity of toothpaste, tooth decay has not decreased.

If the body has a calcium shortage, it dissolves teeth and bones and takes the needed calcium. The body takes from the teeth and bones because the blood calcium should be maintained at a constant level. This is crucially important for the body's cells, blood coagulation, and many other purposes. For many years, European women would say that each time a woman bore a baby she lost one tooth. Scientists laughed at this as an old wives tale, but now highly developed machines clearly show that the body takes out calcium from bones and teeth if necessary. Once the body gets enough calcium, it puts back the calcium into the bones. However, once teeth are destroyed, they never come back.

Bone Loss

Osteoporosis is a big problem for American women. This is not a new disease, having occurred in European countries but rather rarely and exclusively among affluent elderly women, and was called Dowager's hump. Now some twenty million people are suffering from osteoporosis in the United States alone. Painful bone destruction makes people crippled and finally even death results. The causes are said to be calcium deficiency, estrogen trouble, not enough exercise, etc. No good treatment has been established. Clearly, excess sugar creates osteoporosis. Prevention is easy: just don't eat sugar and other sweets. To stop the pain, do the same. A long time is needed for recovery even after you quit eating sugar, but it is possible.

As evidence, the highest incidence of osteoporosis is among Eskimos. Why? Because they eat sugar. When European explorers went to the arctic zone for the first time, the Eskimos were healthy and strong people with much stamina. Without doctors or hospitals, almost no sick people could be found. They ate mostly fish and animal meat because few other foods grow there. Now they are importing sugar and fruit, which are not suited for the arctic zone. Thus, many things have changed; instead of short-bodied people, they have become taller and are now approaching the world average. But on the other hand, osteoporosis, tuberculosis, and other new diseases are rampant. Sugar makes the body taller, but if people become weaker, it is hard to say that a taller body is desirable.

In the past, the disease known as rickets was thought to be caused by a vitamin D deficiency, including lack of sunshine. However, why don't more people in northern countries or in the polar zones get rickets? Ancient people's problems with rickets were rather rare. Suddenly rickets has become very common since the seventeen century. Clearly it is the excess sugar we are eating that causes calcium and vitamin D deficiencies, and this is now recognized as one of the true causes of rickets.

The Best Sources of Calcium

Calcium should be taken in our food rather than as a supplement. It is one of the most abundant inorganic minerals on the earth. Gypsum, limestone chalk, and marble are calcium compounds. Plants take it from the soil, and animals eat the plants to get their calcium. Organic calcium that comes from living things, especially that from plants, is the ideal form for the human body; mineral supplements of inorganic calcium can form kidney stones and calcium deposits in the joints, so they are better avoided. The best and most concentrated sources of calcium are the sea vegetables (some kinds have up to fourteen times as much as cow's milk per serving) and many different kinds of seeds and nuts. Sesame seeds are very high in calcium, as are almonds. While dairy products also have calcium, for many reasons it is best to avoid them in our daily diet and get calcium directly from vegetal sources.

Eating Our Own Tissues

You don't have to be an octopus; the human body also eats itself. This is a normal function of the body and is always occurring naturally. During fasting or starvation the body loses weight. This means that the body is using its own tissues for nutrition. This process is performed by the body in a very biologically economical way, for the body knows what is more important and what is less important. It uses the tissues which are less important such as fat deposits, diseased tissues, and abnormal growth faster than normal tissues.[5] The important organs are reserved until the last stage.

Many people recover perfectly even from severe starvation after they eat. Weight loss from an extremely high fever is also usually replaced. But if anyone eats excess sugar while having protein shortage, this is completely different, although it looks similar to malnutrition. The symptoms appear in many different forms: fatigue, weight loss, slow movement, anemia, dizziness, cold body, nervousness, low blood pressure, coarse skin, loss of hair, poor vision, cyanosis, and others. If one takes sugar continuously, symptoms of hypoglycemia may likely develop.

If powerful disease-causing microbes invade such a body, local-ized destruction in important parts of the body occurs. Polio myeli-tis is one example. It has been said that the polio virus is living in the intestines of many people, in the soil, and everywhere through-out the world, but only a few people are infected severely, losing nerve cells, muscle tissues, etc. It appears that the body is eating its own tissues or that sugar is eating the muscles. These kinds of losses are hard to recover and are often permanent. Many kinds of atrophy, muscular dystrophy, multiple sclerosis, arthritis, and many others are related to excess sugar-eating. These are real degenerative diseases.

Malnutrition

Malnutrition means a total shortage of food or that some nut-rients are missing. In this affluent society, malnutrition is coming not from food shortages, but from sugar-eating. We can think of nutrition loss from two sides. If we buy whole grains, the price is cheap and much nutrition is there. But many people buy candy, cakes, and ice cream, which cost many times more than grain. Even the poorest people buy sweet foods and then complain about a money shortage. This is at the same time a money loss and a nutrition loss. And the damage to the body is much greater.

Sugar and Blood Diseases

Other diseases brought about by excess consumption of sugar and lack of protein are hemophilia and other bleeding disorders, both internally and externally, in which normal clotting or coagula-tion of the blood does not occur. These clotting factors are all mainly protein and require calcium ions to work. Why do some people lack these coagulative factors? This is primarily a salt, cal-cium, phosphorous, and protein deficiency, but even if these peo-ple eat meat or other high protein foods, their condition does not change. For a long time they have probably been taking excessive amounts of sugar, which melted the calcium, the body tissues, and the protein stored in the muscles. Sugar acts as an anti-coagulation factor as a sulfate-containing polysaccharide.[6] As long as they continue to eat sugar, this situation cannot be reversed. Any protein they eat to compensate for the deficiency only produces effects like bed sweating, fever, excessive and uncontrollable sexual desire, and more discharge of mucus or sputum from the windpipe.

The calcium deficiency resulting from excess sugar will also worsen any problems with blood coagulation. Calcium pills or injections can control this temporarily, but salt is critical, for without it the body cannot keep calcium in solution. Even with inherited factors, good quality salt in the diet can help to control this condition. Tuberculosis is often cured without antibiotics this way. Sanatoriums located near the salt water ocean have had better results than the same facilities in mountain areas. The salt in the air helps to heal the lungs, and the sunshine helps to offset calcium deficiencies by providing vitamin D. If the patients stop taking sugar, the good effects can be dramatic.

As mentioned earlier, calcium in its inorganic forms, such as gypsum, limestone, marble, oyster shell or egg shell, may form calcium deposits in the joints or painful stones in the kidneys or other organs. I recommend the organic calcium in greens, root vegetables, seeds, sea vegetables, and nuts. Calcium is always readily available in foods.

Hemophilia

About 50 percent of the people classified as hemophiliacs are so by heredity, while the other half show no evidence of inherited factors. Hemophilia is known as the bleeding disease because the patient does not have normal clotting abilities in the blood and runs a high risk of bleeding to death. Now hemophiliacs are in the AIDS high-risk group through the use of Plasma Factor VIII, a blood-clotting agent made up of blood from thousands of donors. Unfortunately, one or more of these donors contributed the AIDS virus to this supply.

Hemophilia is not a new disease, but in the past it was very rare. The first person modern medicine recognized as having hemophilia was Queen Victoria of England in the last century. Since that time, patients appeared in European royal families so that it has been called the Royal Disease.

The cause is thought to be hereditary, carried with the sex chromosomes. But still there is some question. The antecedents of Queen Victoria did not show any signs of hemophilia. So, some scholars think that the mutation of genes occurred within Victoria herself. Probably this is right, as she consumed a lot of sugar.

Now in the United States alone there are an estimated hundred thousand hemophiliacs. Since there are not many European royal families in this country, factors other than heredity are clearly more important. If sweet foods, even sweet fruits, are avoided for one year, it is possible for a hemophiliac's bleeding to cease; then, the dangerous Plasma Factor VIII injections are not needed.

In the past, one of the great riddles for physiologists was why hemophilia did not exist among many women. Here is my theory: A million or so years ago when our ancestors began eating fruits, the taste was so tempting that many of them ate too much. As fruits have a high proportion of sugar (fructose), hemophilia, or non-coagulation of the blood, developed in both men and women; this was caused by the negative effects of sugar on the blood-clotting process – protein depletion plus calcium and salt deficiencies, as we have seen. Since a woman has a natural bleeding period, however, she would soon die or be unable to bear children if her body lost much of its power to clot the blood. Some developed stronger abilities of blood coagulation than others and survived and increased, even if they did eat fruit, while the weaker ones died. This process continued over thousands of generations and hence there were few women with hemophilia. But now, with the great increase in sugar consumption, things have changed.

Sugar and AIDS

Two types of bodies, obese and thin, can result from heavy sugar consumption. If a person gets enough protein and eats much sugar, this can create an obese body. If a person has a protein shortage and consumes excess sugar, then the body can become thin, losing much nutrition and weight. People who are slim-bodied for this reason are weak against infections of the respiratory organs such as the common cold, flu, tuberculosis, and pneumonia. These are airborne infections which are highly contagious. Also, the brain and nervous systems of such people are weak.

New AIDS research shows that the AIDS virus can attack the brain and nervous system directly before destroying white blood cells. This is the most difficult problem because the brain damage is said to be mostly permanent. Opportunistic infections of AIDS are mainly *Pneumocystis carinii* pneumonia followed by tuberculosis and *Candida*. Other fungal infections are also common.

These kinds of infections have a relationship to meat-eating, since meat-eating produces acid blood, which provides good nutrition for the invading microbes. But sugar has a stronger relationship to brain and lung troubles. People who are playing the meat and sugar game are susceptible to many diseases.

All sugar is of plant origin. If eaten in excess and on a regular basis, all sources of sugar - vegetables, fruits, various syrups (extracts of corn, maple syrup, barley, rice, or other grains), and honey - can cause similar degenerative effects as I have explained in this chapter. To me, the order of this is as follows: Honey is the strongest, then table sugar, then dried fruits, then fresh fruits. Honey is a simple form of sugar, but is very concentrated even when it is raw and completely natural. Do not deceive yourself that, because honey or any other sweet food is natural, it is safe.

Many people in the world are vegetarians, but there are few fruitarians. Saccarians cannot exist, for no one can survive by eating only sugar. Even honeybees cannot live on honey alone; they also eat pollen (protein) and salt. But the longtime habit of eating sugar is very difficult to break. Many people have told me during the past forty-five years that it would be better to die than to stop eating sugar. That is a sad but free choice for anyone to make. For an adult without AIDS or any degenerative illness who wants to eat some amount of sugar, I suggest a four-month blood cleansing period with no sugar, then a maximum of two ounces per day in diluted forms – mixed in with flour products, beverages, etc. A high percentage of sugar in any given food is more damaging than a food with a low (less than 5 percent) sugar content which converts more slowly to calories. This is less dangerous but also less sweet. In the case of cancer, the chemical sweeteners are the most dangerous, but for AIDS, an FDA-approved artificial sweetener is possibly better than sugar.

Chapter 5

Grains

If meat and sugar are omitted from the diet, then what foods are to be recommended for our daily lives? From my observations, from history, and from the evidence of our ancestors' evolutionary process we can say that whole grains are the proper and best life-sustaining foods for humans.

Staple Food

Throughout most of the world, grains are the major staple of the diet, with small amounts of other foods revolving around them. There is rice in Asia; bulghur wheat in the Middle East; pasta (from wheat) in Italy; kasha and black bread in Russia; oat, wheat, and rye breads and cereals in Europe; and corn (maize) in Mexico and other Central and South American countries. As a principal food grains contain the most balanced proportion of necessary nutrients – protein, fat, carbohydrates, vitamins, and minerals – the best quality of each for the body's use. Grains contain no harmful or toxic materials and as such are suitable for eating always and in generous amounts.

It is very interesting that wheat, rice, corn, millet, rye, oats, barley, and sorghum all belong to the same botanical family, Gramineae or Poales (often called the grain or grass family, including more than six thousand different species), all having similar character and nutrients. The fact that all humans eat the seeds of this family of plants is not just a coincidence, for these foods are necessary and designed for us.

Many kinds of animals have come from the same ancestors after the long process of evolution. The body of each species of animal has adapted to certain ideal foods such that now different animals have their own special foods, often within a rather narrow range. Rabbits and giraffes, for instance, eat grass and leaves almost exclusively. These are herbivores. Lions, tigers, and cats, the carnivores, eat other animals. Humans, who eat both plants and animal meat, are considered omnivores. Omni in Latin means all or everything, but this description is not quite accurate; we cannot eat soil as the earthworms do, or wood like the termites. There are limitations for us as well. However, humans are highly developed and can eat from a wide range of foods. This is a great advantage for human survival and people can live almost everywhere on the earth's surface, from the arctic to the tropics. The diet of the Eskimo has traditionally consisted of about 90 percent fish and animal meat; they may eat more meat than carnivorous animals, yet they continue to survive and grow in the arctic. Other groups are vegetarian, some eating plant foods exclusively. But if we were to apply any one diet, either vegetarian or carnivorous, to everyone, we would have many problems. To understand why grains are specially suited to humans, we can again state the conclusion first: the human body developed by eating grains, so these are still the most harmonious foods for us.

Human Evolution and Civilization

Our relationship with grains goes back to about fifty million years ago when the newly established grass family spread over the world, and when our ancestors were still a kind of rodent and probably ate and stored grains in a manner similar to certain rodents of today. About ten million years ago our ancestors were a kind of primate. Before the hands developed, they stood on two legs to eat grains from the top areas of plants and thus the legs became stronger. As the legs became stronger, the front limbs developed into hands. These hands and legs are unique in comparison with other bipedal animals. Birds, monkeys, and apes can walk short distances on two legs but this is not their main mode of locomotion.

How our ancestors acquired this bipedal ability is an interesting subject and many different theories have been offered. Some of these interesting opinions are: to hold stones or tools, for making tools, to make the body appear much larger to predators, to carry infants (especially for mothers), or to protect the body from getting cold and wet on the snowy ground.

There is no way to prove these speculations, but each is reasonable and probably contributed to a certain degree. Still, this explanation is not perfect. The most important motive for animal activity is always to eat food. Our ancestors were no exception. They stood up and ate, and trained their bodies as a result. The best evidence is found in the remaining teeth of ancient skeletons of our ancestors. They have developed molars and large jaw bones which show their main food was grain and that they chewed their food very well.

If we ate nothing but vegetables or fruits, within a week, or a month at the most, we would be having problems. These kinds of foods are lacking in proteins and fats as well as vitamins A, B, D, E, and others. But if we eat grains, we have no problem. And if we add small amounts of beans, seeds, and vegetables to the grain, we can sustain health for our whole life. In Asian countries many people are following such a diet for reasons of economy or by religious teachings.

Archaeological research shows that early prototypes of cultivated wheat existed in the Paleolithic Age.[1] If this is true, it would date wheat at about two million years ago. Crude milling implements have been found dating back seventy-five thousand years, as well as fertilized maize (corn) pollen, estimated to be eighty thousand years old. The oldest known ruins of human civilization were discovered in Southwest Asia, believed to be about nine thousand years old. To maintain the large population of ancient cities, the biggest problems were transportation and the storage of food. At that time, people in settled areas were eating primarily wheat; vegetables and fruits were available in smaller amounts, on occasion. Rice was cultivated in Southeast Asia at least five thousand years before Christ.

Grains and the Brain

While these physical changes were happening, there was an unexpected big change: the development of the brain. The eating of good quality, complex carbohydrates was an important factor in this development, since these foods provided a steady, even supply of glucose for the brain's functioning. The other major factor that aided the brain's development was the increased capacity of the lungs when man stood up. This allowed more oxygen to be taken in and provided the brain with a better supply. The brain uses 20 percent or more of the body's total supply of blood sugar and is the largest consumer of oxygen in the body – 25 to 33 percent of the total intake. When these primitive humans began stretching their arms out to the sides, the lungs, and subsequently the brain, developed even more. The discovery of fire gave man the ability to transmute foods by cooking them, thereby unlocking the molecular structure of carbohydrates and making their absorption more efficient. The development of the brain made humans unique among all the animal species.

At a certain point in time our ancestors began and continued to cultivate grains. Up to the present day grains are produced in great abundance. All over the world we are still cultivating mainly grains, as shown in Figure 3. This is set by natural human intelligence, not as a proportion designed at a desk. About 42.4 percent, or almost one-half, of all food production is in grains. The next highest is

Figure 3. World Production of Food Plants[2]

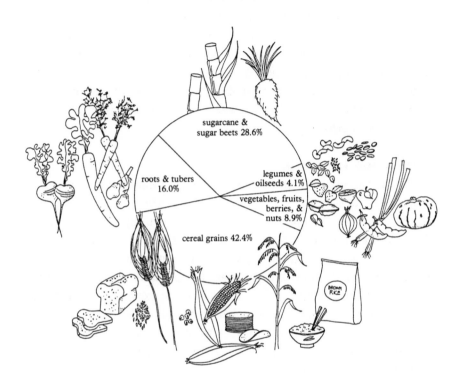

sugar, then roots and tubers (including potatoes), then vegetables, and lastly fruits. Seeds and legumes are produced only in small amounts. Domestic animals also like to eat grains and about 15 percent of grain production goes to animal feed.

Many different grains are grown everywhere under various conditions of climate and geography, but any kind of grain makes an excellent and delicious food. Grains can be eaten whole, as a cereal meal, or ground into flour (or sprouted and ground) and made into breads, casseroles with vegetables, and so on. What one can do with grains is limited only by the creativity and imagination of the cook. Beer, sake and many kinds of alcoholic drinks are brewed from grains. From this long history of eating grains, our ancestors learned to make many preparations. It is said that wheat makes six hundred different foods. No other single food can make such a variety.

Grains are seeds, but they have a unique character in that they are both fruit and seed fused perfectly yet maintaining the appearance of seeds. This is probably why they have such a complicated composition, containing so many nutrients such as protein, fat, carbohydrates, minerals, and vitamins.

With the coming of the Ice Age there was a food shortage and man started to hunt and to eat meat. Plants could not grow in the ice and many people moved to the tropical zone for humans are not hairy and could not survive without fire. Our ancestors were forced to eat anything they could find, any kind of animal, in order to survive. Starvation was a great disadvantage to the human race but still our ancestors found some advantages. They acquired an increased ability to adapt to a variety of foods.

But they did not give up eating grains, for the body was already adapted to them. This is very important. Each animal developed differently due mainly to the food they ate. The human body developed in ways best suited for obtaining, eating, and digesting this particular food. For example, we have twenty grinder teeth with thick enamel covers and our saliva contains large amounts of enzymes designed to break down the carbohydrates in grains. Our long intestines show that our body is similar to that of the herbivorous animals, and our stomach does not secrete the quantity of hydrochloric acid needed for the digestion of large amounts of meat.

If the food is changed, the body starts to develop toward a different way. This change does not occur suddenly as evolution is a very slow process. In this changing process many individuals who are unable to adapt to the new food die. Those who are able to adapt produce offspring and increase. Thus change may occur in two opposite ways, but the stability of the species is primarily important. If too big a change occurs, the result will not be human beings anymore.

To establish stability, we need the stability of foods. So, to stay healthy and prevent diseases and birth defects, it would be good to eat grains as our ancestors did for millions of years. Just two hundred years ago, whole grains were a big part of the human diet. In European countries, the majority of the population ate peasant food, almost all whole grains.[3] Even bread was not popular except among city people. No individual house had an oven or a grain mill. The peasants were healthier than city people and raised more children. Civilizations could not have persisted without the flow of healthier migrants from the countryside to the city.

What The Teeth Tell Us

Archaeologists have discovered bones considered to be early human which have been dated as old as 4.5 million years. At that point in time the body was still slightly curved like an ape's, but what is most important is the teeth, and since these were molars, these bones are considered to be of our human ancestors. The molars are the grinding teeth that each of us have to this day.

The molars are our most developed teeth, twenty in number, tightly covered with thick enamel and designed specifically for grinding grains. The four canines are for eating meat, but compared to the canine teeth of other animals, they are small and imperfectly shaped, similar to those of herbivorous animals. The eight front incisors are for cutting vegetables and fruits.

After our ancestors developed hands, they used them for picking food and putting it in their mouths. The prominent mouth and teeth became useless and the shape of the jaw bones changed from a tunnel-shaped arch to more of a rainbow shape. This is also unique among animals.

Modern people's teeth show some signs of deterioration. The

Figure 4. Comparisons of Jaws and Teeth

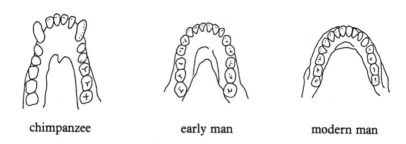

chimpanzee   early man   modern man

significant one is the losing of four molars due to lack of chewing. These teeth are called wisdom teeth because they come in after the body grows up. Some people never have them, while others have much trouble with pain or not enough space in the jaw bones, etc. Often they are extracted, hopefully without the person losing wisdom.

From the total of thirty-two teeth, Dr. Sagen Ishizuka (an army physician in Japan, late 1800s) suggested a good proportion of different foods.[4] The four canines constitute 12.5 percent of the thirty-two teeth and their primitive shape indicates this percentage as the maximum proportion of animal food. The eight incisors make up about 25 percent, so this is the proportion of vegetables and fruits that should be eaten. The twenty molars make up 62.5 percent of our teeth; grains should roughly equal this proportion of our total food intake.

This is reasonable, but in my opinion this recommendation is only for healthy people. Sick people need to eat a more vegetarian diet.

Expendable and Durable Nutrients

We need a good proportion of nutrients in each meal. Sugar contains almost no fiber. Meat contains small percentages of undigestible substances, but almost no carbohydrates or fiber. For many years dietary fiber was thought to be a needless substance, for our body cannot break down fiber for nutrition. Later discoveries have shown it to be very important for good elimination of food wastes; this, in turn, helps in the prevention of cancer, heart attack, and other abnormal conditions. Animal fats can be used by the body for fuel, but it is now widely accepted that these are danger- ous for our health in large amounts. Both sugar and meat are extremely unbalanced foods. If we eat these foods in good propor- tion, we can balance sugar and protein, or fuel material and body- building material, but there is no way to supply enough minerals, vitamins, or dietary fiber. So, we have another problem: how do we determine a good proportion of sugar and meat?

Cell-building material is mainly protein, a durable nutrient, one we can use for a long time once we have built up the body. When the cells become old, they are destroyed and replaced by new ones, but amino acids from old cells are reused for new cells. Protein also can be used for fuel, but this is as a substitute and is not its most economical use. At the end of the nineteenth century, the famous physiologist Carl von Voit researched human nutritional needs and calculated the daily protein requirement to be about 107 grams (four ounces). At the time this was widely accepted, but today new researchers calculate a smaller amount: W.C. Rose, 18 gm and Hegsted, 10 gm. The World Health Organization tentatively fixed the amount at 37 gms.[5] However, compared with the nutrients necessary for fuel, these amounts are relatively small – about 2 to 17 percent of carbohydrate intake.

Other durable nutrients are minerals, important building mate- rials for bones, teeth, the brain, and other specialized cells. Cal- cium, phosphorus, magnesium, sodium, chlorine, sulfur, and po- tassium are called major essential minerals, even though the daily requirement for them is calculated in milligrams (1/1000 of a gram). About thirty-seven other essential minerals have been researched and recommended, but exactly how many kinds we need is not known. Our daily need for these minerals (known as trace elements) is calculated in micrograms (1/1,000,000 of a gram). Then, too, certain minerals are used as expendable nutrients for the proper functioning of the body. So our thinking must be flexible, as we cannot say exactly that nutrients are used just as durable or expendable materials; for example, a remarkable amount of chloride is also used as expendable nutrition. Such small amounts of these kinds of nutrients are crucially important for maintaining our good health. The problem is that no one knows the exact kinds we need, and in what amounts. These are always changing with new research.

Grains and Longevity

Those races of people around the world who are known for their vitality and longevity, such as the Hunzas of Northwest Pakistan, the Vilcabambas of the Ecuadorean Andes, and the Georgian mountain people of the Russian Caucasus, all have similar dietary patterns and ways of life. For these people, grain is the staple food, supplemented by beans and locally grown vegetables and fruits in season.

Thus a low protein, low fat, no refined foods or sugars, and high complex carbohydrate diet, such as I am recommending in this book, has been instrumental in keeping these people remarkably disease-free, fit, and active well past the age of 100, and in some cases as long as 150 years.[6]

David Davies, a British doctor, has researched long-lived people of the Andes mountains. By consulting church records of births and deaths he found many of these people lived more than 120 years. He also found that a hundred-year-old man could father a baby by a young woman the age of his grandchildren. Women's lives were found to be somewhat shorter than men's by 10 or 20 years. Menstruation usually continued until after the age of sixty and there were no unpleasant symptoms to accompany menopause. The foods of these people, like the Hunzas, is almost entirely grains

Figure 5. Proportions of Major Cereal Crops[7]

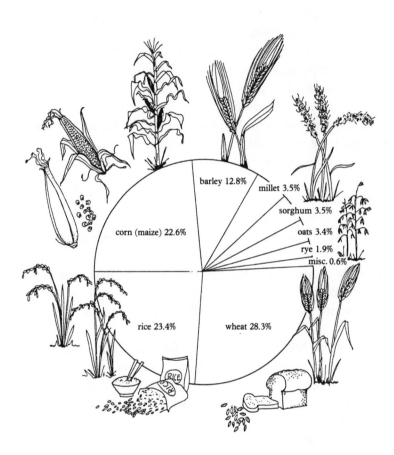

along with some vegetables and fruits (99 percent vegetarian).

Refined Grains

White rice had been known in many countries from ancient times, but much labor was needed for the refining process and only royal families and aristocrats could eat white rice occasionally. Other people almost never ate it before the invention of the milling machine. During the middle of the 19th century Asian people learned about white flour and white bread and they tried to apply the same process to rice. They imported milling machines from Western countries and began milling rice.

The result was an outbreak of the disease beri-beri, originating in the large cities among people who ate white rice. At that time about half a million people died every year in Asian countries. The first symptoms of beri-beri are fatigue, dullness, and loss of appetite. The next stage is numbness in the muscles or body pain without any specific reason. Sometimes the legs become swollen and in other cases the muscles shrink. Other symptoms are heart palpitation, weakened sight, shortness of breath, and in advanced cases, the body can become paralyzed and finally the patient dies of heart failure. The disease pattern looks similar to the plague and doctors suspected some kind of bacteria as the cause. However, the causative agent has never been discovered.

Christiaan Eijkman, a Dutch physician living in Java, found that chickens fed white rice contracted a disease similar to beri-beri, while those fed brown (unrefined) rice did not. Also, those that already had the disease who were fed brown rice recovered. He understood that something was missing from white rice in 1897. In 1911, Casimir Funk isolated crystals with vitamin B-complex activity and this was the first discovery of the vitamin. Many B vitamins and other important nutrients are stored in the germ of the rice. When rice is milled or polished, the grain loses the whole germ.

It was then understood why the disease attacked mainly city people, because they adopted white rice immediately. The rural areas did not use the milling machine so early and the diet of the peasants included other whole grains such as barley, wheat, oats, and buckwheat. Now, this vitamin is called thiamin or vitamin B_1 and many other vitamins have also been identified.

Asian people began taking vitamins for the prevention and cure of beri-beri and now they are enriching the white rice with vitamins. It seems that the problem is completely resolved, but actually it is not. Still in Japan about twenty thousand people annually are dying from this disease despite the developed vitamin B treatment. If people would eat whole grain rice instead of white rice with vitamin B_1 added, and would quit eating sugar, beri-beri could be avoided.

A similar problem is pellagra, a niacin or vitamin B_3 deficiency, which also starts with fatigue, loss of appetite, weak muscles, and indigestion. Accompanying symptoms are various skin eruptions and small ulcers, diarrhea, and nervous disorders. The disease is found mostly in India, the near East, and African countries among people who have newly adopted corn as the staple food, yet native American people who have been eating corn since ancient times seldom have such troubles. Corn is covered by a coarse, hard skin, and machines now remove this skin easily to make corn starch, corn flour, cornmeal, etc. The corn germ contains niacin, vitamin E, and protein, but in the refining process the germ and its nutrients are lost. Again, the problem is in refining the whole grain.

Yet another problem is created by the grinding of grains. Almost all Americans eat white bread made with white flour. The wheat is not only ground but also most of it is bleached in the process. Wheat is a good grain and, even after refining, does not cause severe malnutrition diseases like corn and rice do, but fiber loss is inevitable. As a result, some bakeries have started adding wooden pulp instead of wheat fiber to make high fiber bread. This does not seem like the right thing to do.

The bigger problem is with the storing of white flour, or any grain, once it has been ground. The grain starts to deteriorate immediately. The enzymes inside the grain remain dormant as long as the grain is whole. Once the grain is broken the enzymes start working and cause damage. Also, many kinds of bugs are attracted to flour, much more so than to whole grains.

The quality of flour changes quickly by the process of oxidation.

Once ground, any kind of grain should be used immediatley. This is difficult with the modern commercial system because any flour you buy in the stores is already very old. Thus it is good to have your own grain mill and to make your own flour. Do not store flour more than one month.

The refining of grains destroys the balance of the nutrients. Modern nutritional research seems to be very developed, but still there are plenty of unknown minor nutrients and enzymes. We need to go back to eating whole grains.

The Most Successful Plant

If human beings are the most successful of all the animals in the world, and if eating grain has largely made this possible, then the grain family is the most successful among the plants. Our ancestors were fortunate to have chosen these plants for their food, since they grow almost everywhere – from the tropics to the arctic, from the ocean shore to the highest mountains like the Alps or the Himalayas, in deserts and in water. A very large proportion of the earth's surface is covered by human populations and these plants.

Usually the plants of the grain family are small in size, but not always. For example, the bamboo can be six inches in diameter and grow to a height of 140 feet. Never have any poisonous substances been reported in the stalks or seeds of these grass family plants; only on rare occasions do new sprouts from the roots contain some poison. This means that these plants are very important food for livestock and birds. The seeds of the bamboo plant are delicious and nutritious, but hard to collect. We can only gather the seeds from the bamboo every sixty years. They so resemble rice grains that Asian peoples call it wild rice. After the bamboo plant dies, the roots go on living so the following spring they can sprout again and the plant can continue to flourish. Many kinds of bamboo shoots are edible. They have a strong taste, but with suitable cooking make delicious vegetable dishes. Fibers of bamboo are so strong that carbonized bamboo fiber was used by Thomas Edison to make the filament of the first electric lamp.

Sugar cane is another member of this same family. There is no reason for us to exclude the sugar cane as food. If you live in areas which produce it, cut it fresh, chew it well, perhaps one thousand times, and swallow the sweet juice and the fiber together as our ancestors probably did, no harm is done. If we add sugar cane to the list of the world's grain production we find that 80 percent of all human food comes from the grain families of plants. Before the cultivation of sugar spread all over the world, people probably cultivated other grains at about this percentage.

Buckwheat, quinoa, and amaranth are not grains but seeds; however, they are often used as grain substitutes because of their similarity to grains. In some areas of the world it is difficult to grow grains and so it is good to cultivate this kind of food. Cows mainly eat this family of plants, so milk and beef are made from grass. Chickens eat mostly corn, so eggs and chicken meat are made from corn. If one eats eggs and meat, then the body is indirectly of grass origin. The contribution of this family of plants for human life is surely great.

Chapter 6

Beans, Seeds, and Nuts

Next to grains, beans are the most nutritionally balanced food for humans. There are many varieties of beans, but they all belong to one family, the Leguminosae, or the Fabaceae, commonly known as the bean family.

Beans, like grains, were cultivated by our ancestors at an early date. Some bean and pea seeds were discovered in an ancient cave in southern India, shown by carbon dating to be about ten thousand years old.[1] Beans have been an important human food for a long time, sometimes used as a staple food in many areas of the world.

Fat, protein, and carbohydrate are the important nutrients in beans, and generally the fat and protein content is very high. Soybeans contain about 34 percent protein in their dry form. Cooked soybeans contain about 14 percent protein. Meat, considered the highest protein food, contains about 16 to 20 percent. Peanuts, green peas, and other beans are also high in protein – about 20 to 28 percent (raw) – so beans and animal foods have a similar protein content. However, we will see that the character of beans is much different than that of meat.

We know that animals cannot manufacture protein, that protein synthesis is a function of plants and microbes. So it is not strange that beans are high in protein; it is interesting that they can produce such large amounts of it.

Protein is differentiated from other nutrients by its nitrogen content. Nitrogen is abundant in the atmosphere, forming about 80 percent of the air's gases. But nothing can change this abundant gas to the liquid form needed by plants for protein synthesis except microbes or lightning. The bean's special ability to create protein is in its symbiotic relationship with certain bacteria capable of converting nitrogen gas into nitrates and nitrites. Beans form nodes along their roots in which nitrifying bacteria can thrive and increase. That is why beans are self-sufficient nitrogen fertilizers.

Beans are used for extracting oil, as their oil content is also high. Peanuts probably contain the most oil, up to 47 percent by weight. The liquid form of fat at room temperature is called oil, an almost unsaturated fatty acid of better quality than animal fat or saturated fatty acids.

Many researchers have already written about the harmful effects of fat, so here is just one simple example. In wintertime, frostbite is more common in women and children than men. We saw in our discussion of sugar that women and children normally tend to eat more sugar than men do. We also know that animal fat is found in solid form at room temperature. If one eats fat and sugar, the sugar reduces blood circulation and the body temperature in the extremities, the fingers, toes, and ears, is lowered; fat coagulates in these areas, leading to frostbite. The liquid form of vegetable oil, however – such as the oils derived from soybeans, corn, cotton seeds, and other plant foods – will not coagulate except in extremely cold weather. Vegetable oil is soft and flows smoothly through the bloodstream, but animal fat is not smooth even at body temperature. Cholesterol also exists with fat. This leads to trouble in the form of heart disease and high blood pressure.

The skin of beans is even tougher than that of grains. This means that the fiber content is also high. Many people remove the skin from peanuts (which are actually beans, not nuts) or green peas, for example, but it is good to include the skins (not the pods). Peanut skins alone have a peculiar taste, but if we make peanut butter with the skins included, the taste is better and there will be no burning sensation in the stomach. Also, it is best not to add sugar or honey to peanut butter. The fiber content of beans is good for alleviating constipation, so the skins should be used.

Beans are also high in calcium and other minerals; they are usually lacking in vitamin C, but sprouts made from beans are rich in this vitamin and can substitute well for vegetables. Before storage techniques were developed for vegetables, bean sprouts were an important food on long sea journeys. In wintertime, wherever fresh vegetables are not available, beans can be very useful for making sprouts.

If a food is high in protein and fat, it usually means that it is lower in carbohydrates. For this reason beans do not make the best staple for humans. Some starchy foods must be added to complement a bean-centered diet such as potatoes, yams, or other high carbohydrate foods. People seem to know this intuitively or through experimentation, for beans have almost always been combined with grains.

The world production of beans is about 4 percent of all agricultural crops produced, compared to 45 percent for grains.[2] Thus, bean production is about 10 percent that of grains, suggesting that it is good to eat this same proportion, about ten to one. Many different cultures have developed their own combinations. Corn (maize) with pinto beans has been a traditional combination used in Mexico for many centuries; soybeans and rice in Asia; lentils and wheat in the Near East; chapatis (made with wheat) and chickpeas for the long-lived Hunza people of Pakistan. The favorite American combination seems to be bread and peanut butter.

The Soybean Connection

Soybeans constitute about 55 percent of the total bean production, so we can say it is the most common of all the beans; the

United States produces about 60 percent of the world's production, but many people do not know what the soy or soya bean is. It arrived in the United States in 1804 via Asia and Europe: the Midwest, with its favorable climate, has become the world's largest producer. As we have seen, the soybean is composed of about 34 percent protein, 18 percent oil, and 33 percent carbohydrates, plus minerals – especially phosphorus and potassium – and vitamins.

In Asian countries it is rare to eat the soybean just simply cooked; it is almost always eaten after it has undergone some fermentation process, such as we find in traditional Oriental foods like miso, natto, and tempeh, or shoyu (soy sauce). The word shoyu is a Japanese word that was adapted in Western countries to soy to denote the Japanese soya sauce. Through microbial action the fermentation process serves to break down the protein into its component amino acids. We can compare this process to the feeding of soybeans to cattle, which are then served as meat.

Even if the soybean looks the same after fermentation, in quality it is not. In order to make miso, a special yeast, *Aspergillus oryzae* (a green mold of the same genus as penicillin), is cultivated on the grain of choice (rice, wheat, or barley) and then mixed with the soybeans, while in the production shoyu, *Aspergillus sojae* is used.

A relatively new type of soyfood, tofu, readily available in most supermarkets, has become quite popular in this country. In the West there are not many foods like tofu, which is kept in cold water and can be eaten cooked or raw (it has already been cooked during processing). Tofu is made by extracting the protein and combining it with nigari, a natural coagulent made from sea water. It is a good substitute for meat because it is a high-protein food; however, it is hard to say that it is a health food since much of the fiber is removed and thus is a kind of refined food. I have known of some undesirable side-effects from eating an excess of tofu and other bean foods, including a higher incidence of symptoms of goiter and swollen joints. In general it is good to be moderate with the intake of beans and bean products. Asians eat tofu frequently, but in limited amounts.

Often I have talked about troubles caused by excess tofu-eating and have had strong opposition in Japan. But, in this country I have not met much opposition to this viewpoint, as the scientific research in the United States is ahead of Japan's. I also feel that soy milk, like tofu, should be used with caution. Soy milk can be given to babies, but it can never be a substitute for mother's milk. If breast milk is not sufficient, cow's milk is better than soy milk.

Around the beginning of this century in the United States, especially in the Great Lakes region, goiter was almost an epidemic. Scientists and doctors researched the cause and discovered that in this area the soil was lacking in iodine; even the vegetables growing there lacked it. Large doses of iodine were given to goiter patients in 1924 and within twenty-five years it had all but disappeared. People thought that science was great. Strangely enough, though, some people showed similar symptoms from overdoses of iodine. Both an excess and a shortage of iodine causes trouble. Iodine is taken from seaweed, so if these patients had been eating seaweed they may have been able to avoid the disease. At that time in exactly the same area, soybean cultivation had increased markedly. The people who lived there did not know the traditional Eastern way, so they just cooked and ate soybeans in large amounts. At the same time they also increased their consumption of sugar. The harmful side-effects of sugar and soybeans taken together are very strong. There were more cases of goiter among women, since, as we said earlier, women tend to eat more sugar.

Some toxic reactions to and toxic substances in beans have been identified scientifically and these are: trypsin inhibition, cyanogenetic glucosides, saponins, alkaloids, goitrogenic factors, hemagglutinins, etc. These also can be used for some medicinal purposes, but if we eat large amounts of beans for a long period of time, undesirable side-effects manifest. A good way to remove these toxins is to cook the beans well by boiling or steaming for a long time or roasting them before cooking. Cooking beans with seaweeds is also a good method. With some beans it is good to soak them in water before cooking, discarding the soaking water. Mexican people eat large amounts of pinto beans, but they cook them for a whole day or overnight. This is a good practice. I feel such longtime traditions are great.

Undescended Testes

In the United States about 10 percent of newborn boys have undescended testes. The problem is treated surgically or with hormones. In about 9 percent of these boys the problem is resolved somehow and in most cases without treatment. About 1 percent of adults have this trouble. It causes sterility and a high incidence of other diseases including cancer.

If we can discover the cause of this trouble, then surgery or the undesirable side-effects of hormones can be avoided. From my longtime observations, I am suspicious of the large consumption of peanuts. The United States is one of the largest producers of peanuts and the consumption per capita is much higher than elsewhere in the world.

The testes of all land animals hang down from the body, the only exception being the elephant. Presumably, after the huge reptiles became extinct, the elephant family of animals and the bean family of plants were the most prosperous. Even though elephants eat more grasses today, they still like peanuts.

If human mothers eat a lot of peanuts, more abnormal babies with testical problems are born. After these babies grow up they also favor peanuts. If people eat peanuts and sugar (as in most commercial peanut butter), the troubles are even greater. Much research is needed in this area. I am not saying that peanuts are toxic, but do want to give a warning against the large consumption of this food.

The Positive Side of Beans

Now I must say something about the good side of eating beans, otherwise I am not really being fair to the bean. The *Encyclopedia*

Britannica says that red beans increase white blood cells. Even soybeans, when they have undergone the fermentation process (in miso, for example), possess a wonderful nutritional value. They provide all kinds of essential amino acids and many vitamins and minerals. Most of the vitamin B originally present in beans is lost in the cooking process, but fermented beans contain more.

Recently, the Japanese Cancer Institute reported the preventive effect of miso soup against cancer. Their 260,000 subjects were divided into three groups. One group ate miso soup every day, the second group ate it two to three times a week, while the third group did not eat it at all. After twenty-five years of research, these scholars came to the conclusion that the third group, who had not taken the miso soup, showed a 50 percent higher incidence of cancer than the group who took the miso soup.

Throughout the world the lowest incidence of breast cancer occurs among Japanese women, about 10,000 cases per year reported. Among Americans, about 150,000 new cases are recognized annually. The incidence per capita is almost eight times higher than it is among the Japanese. Why this difference? It is too early to say this is due to miso soup; many kinds of co-factors must be considered. Still, some connection with soy products may be significant.

Here is a mysterious story about soybeans. In a mountainous area of Japan, people had a special folk remedy for painful acute infections in the central area of the face around the nose. This is called the dangerous triangle and the infection is often life-threatening. Modern research shows it is caused by staphylococcus, but these people did not know anything about bacteria. They just experimented and passed the remedy from generation to generation.

As soon as abnormal symptoms appeared they would take three raw, dry, yellow soybeans and chew them well. If the patient thought the beans had a bad taste and spat them out, then a different treatment was needed. If the patient didn't experience a bad taste, then this was indication that it was the right treatment. After swallowing the masticated soybeans and taking a day's rest, the person felt fine. I experienced this trouble and the remedy worked wonderfully for me as well as for several other cases where I recommended it. Today, antibiotics work to cure this trouble, so few cases are seen, but if new strains of bacteria come that resist the antibiotics, we would then have the opportunity to test this treatment. Three grains of raw soybeans are not poisonous.

One of the most common and very important herbs in Oriental medicine is kuzu (kudzu, ko-ken, pueraria thunbergiana). This is a relatively new plant in America. About 120 years ago this plant was a wonderful gift from Japan to make the barren land greener. It is a strong plant and grows well in poor soil. However, too much grew and houses, electrical poles, everything in the Southeast is covered by kudzu. People hate it and are trying to eradicate it. But if Americans understood how to use it, the problem would be solved easily. Kudzu is a member of the bean family and the root can be used for herb tea or the starch may be extracted for food. It is useful in combination with other herbs for fevers, inflammation, tight muscles, muscle pains, to stimulate urination, etc. Eating the starch is helpful in stopping diarrhea. The root is dug out of the ground and chopped into small pieces. This is then dried and used as an herb. The dried root may be pounded to remove the starch. It is interesting to note that if we can find the most suitable ones, nutritionally unbalanced foods can be more effective than the more-balanced grain family for curing diseases caused by an unbalanced condition.

Seeds

The third best group of foods is seeds, and nuts are included here as they are larger single seeds contained in a hard shell. Seeds and nuts occur in many different kinds of plants, and it is interesting that they are botanical end products yet at the same time hold inside themselves the embryos of future plants. For this reason their nutritional content is more complex, containing many varieties of minerals and vitamins. They are especially high in oil and protein.

Probably beans and seeds, including nuts, constituted our ancestors' basic food prior to the development of grains. Many people feel that our ancestors ate mostly fruits as monkeys do, but this is not true. Many scholars agree that the ancestors of monkeys were rodents, who ate seeds, nuts, and grains as well as tree leaves, roots, tubers, and bark and stored these various foods in their nests. So it is likely that our early ancestors stayed in the trees in order to escape predators and so ate some fruits and leaves, but during the daytime usually came down from the trees and ate seeds and nuts which had fallen to the ground.

For body development high protein foods were desirable, as they are for modern-day people, but for brain development more carbohydrates were needed. Our ancestors slowly changed their principal food from seeds to grains. As a result their bodies developed differently from rodents, eventually resulting in the flourishing of today's humankind.

Grains are also seeds. Our ancestors ate mostly this kind of food and their numbers increased all over the world. Many different sources have said such things as, "Seeds are good for the reproductive organs," or "The seeds of plants make human seed." This may sound like folklore, but we hear it also from medical professionals. Dr. W. Devrient of Berlin, for example, wrote an article which claimed that "pumpkin seeds can prevent prostate gland cancer, lessen women's sufferings during menopause, and also increase male potency; these were not all the good effects that came from eating pumpkin seeds."[3] I too think it is reasonable to expect that seeds will have a positive effect on the sex organs. If AIDS is a sex-related disease, then why not try this kind of food? The patient cannot lose by it and seeds (and grains) are far less expensive than meat.

Vitamin E was thought to be an essence of seeds, for wheat germ oil was the first source from which vitamin E was obtained. Other vegetable oils, and all whole raw grains, seeds, and nuts have high concentrations of this vitamin. In experiments, laboratory rats fed with vitamin E showed markedly increased fertility compared to those fed regular food. Because of advertisements from drug companies, the public believed that science had discovered a new aphrodisiac, and pharmacies sold many vitamin E supplements. This was a fad about ten years ago. Unfortunately, this same experiment made on humans did not give such results, but many good effects were found for a number of diseases. Research on vitamin E continued and it was found in butter, eggs, meat and animal organs, avocados, and green vegetables. In the near future another nutrient will be identified from seeds. Vitamins are important elements of nutrition taken in from the outside, and food usually contains enough vitamins for our needs. In special cases vitamin supplements may be helpful. But hormones are produced in the body and should not be taken in from the outside. How can the body produce more hormones? Through chewing grains and seeds very well, as Dr. Devrient also recommended.

Acorns and horse chestnuts contain toxic substances and have a bitter taste. They are usually unfit to eat, but for ancient people in times of famine or crop failure these were important foods. We haven't had such food shortages in a long time, but in future emergencies we may again need to eat such foods. To remove the bitter taste and toxicity, crush the seeds or nuts and soak them in water, changing the water frequently. Within a few days the toxins should be gone and the starch can be prepared. Many kinds of other beans, seeds, and nuts can probably become edible through such a simple process. But how did our ancestors find out whether seeds were edible or toxic? There was only one way – chew it and taste it. If it was unpleasant tasting, they spit it out. If it was swallowed they risked stomach pain, nausia, diarrhea, the loss of sight, hearing, or other body functions. The grain family of plants have no such toxic seeds. This is another important reason our ancestors chose grain for their principal food. It is good to remember this as we enjoy grains, beans, seeds, and nuts.

Potatoes

Usually potatoes are classified as vegetables, but since they are a little different from other vegetables, I will mention them here. Potatoes, tubers, and bulbs are also good foods. They are a rich source of carbohydrates as well as certain vitamins, such as vitamin C. They do not have much protein and fat, so they still should be taken mostly as a side dish, not as the main fare.

The most popular kind of potato is the Idaho or Irish potato. It originally came from the Andes mountains but is now cultivated all over the world. More than half of the potatoes produced are of this variety. The potato forms sprouts which grow to new plants. If they are planted in early spring, the harvest will be ready before the summer. If planted in the summer, they will be ready in the fall. And so the potato became an important food which could be eaten when grains were not yet ready for harvesting, and especially in times of famine. Also, the potato is a high-yielding plant and produces a large amount of calories. For these reasons potato production increased all over the world.

In Europe and America the meat consumption increased at the same time that widespread potato cultivation became popular, so it was often mistakenly thought that the potato is a better food than grains. The real reason for the meat/potato association is that meat, a high-protein, high-fat food, combines well with the high-carbohydrate potato.

In the eighteenth century many Europeans visited Ireland and saw that the Irish were eating a lot of potatoes and that their health was excellent. Potato-eating became very popular on the Continent and was often thought of as a healthy thing to do. With its large amounts of potassium and vitamin C, the potato is a good complement for meat-eaters. If the consumption of meat is reduced, the potato cannot be recommended as a staple food for vegetarians.

The meat-and-potato diet is popular in Germany, but in other countries sugar is rapidly taking the potato's place and potato consumption is slowly declining.

After the Idaho potato the varieties most commonly used are sweet potatoes and yams. These also originated in South America. To be exact, yams are a kind of potato grown only in the tropical zone. In the United States there is no such plant and people use the term yam for a variety of sweet potato which is sweeter-tasting than any other potato. It has a high vitamin A precursor content in the form of carotene, a name derived from the carrot which shares a similar color. If required, our body can convert carotene to vitamin A. This vitamin is important for body growth and other functions, especially eyesight. Night blindness is considered to be caused by a deficiency of vitamin A.

I would like to suggest sweet potatoes as a snack or dessert, especially for children or those who want sweet foods, instead of candies, cakes, or ice cream. It is good to include the skins to prevent constipation and a burning sensation in the stomach.

Chapter 7

Vegetables and Fruits

Besides grains, beans, seeds, and nuts the plant kingdom offers many other valuable foods for our well-being. A simple understanding of the nature of foods is preferable to long listings of vitamin and mineral contents and daily requirements of these and other dietary elements. This is the basic education needed for developing good health and a strong immune system.

A walk through the countryside reveals what an abundant variety of plants there are, many of which are edible in whole or in part. In ancient times this was the standard method of gathering food; thousands of years of experience with the plants in the landscape would dictate which ones were good to eat, which had certain medicinal powers, and so on. Unfortunately this wealth of knowledge about plants has been nearly lost in our times, and since a few plants contain dangerous amounts of toxins, we don't usually go out foraging for wild vegetables and fruits. To avoid mistakes, and for the sake of convenience, we buy the common produce available at the grocery store, usually without giving a thought to where it came from, what its properties are, or even what kind of plant it is. These familiar vegetables and fruits have been cultivated for hundreds and even thousands of generations and have stood the test of time that assures us of a pleasant taste and aroma, beautiful colors, good nutrition, and no poisons.

So many different varieties of vegetables exist that classification into a few basic categories can be helpful. Some are flowers (broccoli, cauliflower, Brussels sprouts, artichokes); some are leaves (lettuce, cabbage); some are stems (celery, asparagus); and some (Swiss chard, spinach, beet greens, etc.) are both leaf and stem. There are roots and tubers (potatoes, onions, beets, carrots, turnips, radishes) and immature seeds (peas, corn, lima beans). Corn, though technically considered a grain, can also be classified as an immature seed. Still other categories are the "unsweet fruits" (eggplant, cucumbers, squash and pumpkins, tomatoes, peppers, and okra). Another important group are the sea vegetables, now becoming very popular for their unique nutritive properties.

One important reason for eating vegetables is that they supply minerals which have been taken up from the soil, although it is now becoming more difficult to get enough minerals from vegetables. The leafy parts of vegetables are the most vital parts; breathing air, synthesizing nutrients, and obtaining water from the roots through the stem. They are always the highest in mineral content and contain many vitamins. Also, the moisture in vegetables is the highest quality water, having been filtered through the long plant bodies. But storage of leafy greens can be a problem for some people, as vegetables will shrink, change color, and lose some enzymes and vitamin C. However, these are still good to eat, if not woody, and the same is true for dried vegetables. Of course, the best way to eat vegetables is fresh from the garden. This may be a little difficult for city people to do, but anyone can cultivate a backyard garden and grow fresh vegetables.

Since roots and tubers store nutrition for the plant, they tend to be high in carbohydrates and they also contain more fat and protein than leaves. The nutritional character of leaves does not vary much, but this is not true of roots. The root vegetables – carrots, radishes, turnips, beets, burdock – all have different colors, different minerals, and different vitamins. For this reason certain root vegetables were traditionally used for medicinal purposes. The most famous example of this is Korean ginseng; other more familiar roots like garlic, burdock, carrots, and leeks are often used in folk remedies. Stem vegetables share the qualities of both leaf and root. The immature seed category is rich in protein and carbohydrates.

Another simple and practical method of classifying vegetables is by color, specifically the colors green, yellow, and white. Green is the color of chlorophyll and denotes the presence of magnesium. Darker shades of green reveal increased levels of calcium and iron. Yellow is the color of carotene. Yellow vegetables are also higher in carbohydrates and phosphorus than other vegetables. Compared to the green and yellow vegetables, white vegetables that grow above the ground contain the least mineral nutrients. Their lack of color shows that they have little or no chlorophyll. But in root vegetables this is not so much the case.

If Idaho potatoes receive sunshine, their skin color will change to green. This means that chlorophyll is present, but this is not a desirable change. The taste changes to what Americans would describe as bitter or harsh, like potash. Not only the green part of the potato but also potato sprouts contain the toxic alkaloid solanine. You must carefully remove and discard these parts. Other problems with the potato are reported from those areas of the world where it is a mainstay of the diet, such as Peru and Ireland; there, the potato is blamed for causing multiple nutritional deficiency diseases. Likely this problem arises not from the potato, but rather the addition of sugar in the diet. This interpretation I believe is verified by the excellent health of their ancestors who ate a diet of potatoes without sugar. But people do not like to think that sugar causes disease, so they blame the potato.

Overall, vegetable foods contain less protein, oil, and carbohydrates and higher levels of minerals, vitamins, and digestive enzymes than other foods. Vegetables neutralize the acids and toxins produced by the consumption of animal foods, thereby cleansing the blood and strengthening many organs that have been weakened by years of eating out of balance.

When choosing vegetables, try to get a variety of the green and yellow types, with some very dark leafy greens whenever possible. Also, be sure to include a little bit of all the various parts of the vegetable – the flower, the stem, the leaves, the roots – into your daily meals. This is the most effective way to cleanse the blood and to build a strong immune system, since vegetables are high in fiber, are excellent for elimination, and contain a variety of nutrients.

Sea Vegetables

Any plant that grows in the sea is a seaweed, botanically known as algae. There are many different names and varieties; it is estimated that there are some two thousand five hundred varieties of marine plants. Among these no toxic seaweeds have ever been found. They can simply be chosen for their flavor and texture. But they are even more exceptional for the nutritional value they provide. We can see how rich they are in minerals, but seaweeds also contain carotene, vitamins D, K, and B_{12}, plus most of the water-soluble vitamins.

With so many varieties of seaweeds to choose from, we can find a wide range in the composition of nutrients. Protein content, for example, may range from 8 to 75 percent; carbohydrates from 4 to 40 percent; lipids from 1 to 86 percent; and ash from 4 to 45 percent. The most widely-used seaweed, kelp (dry kombu), contains about 7 percent protein, 0.5 percent fat, 50 percent carbohydrate, 680 mg of calcium, and 0.062 mg of iodine.[1] Other seaweeds available in markets do not have such a high iodine content, but in regard to other nutrients are almost the same as kelp.

A Japanese doctor by the name of Yuji Kondo studied longevity in a group of Japanese subjects. For over fifty years he seached for long-lived people and studied their diets. He reached the conclusion that what contributed to their long life was a diet consisting mainly of barley, oats, rye, millet, and sorghum, with no white rice; green and yellow vegetables; small whole fish for protein; and

Table 4. Mineral Elements in Dried Seaweed[2]
(Average Analysis, Norwegian Brown Variety)

	Element	Percent		Element	Percent
Ag	Silver	.000004	Mg	Magnesium	.213000
Al	Aluminum	.193000	Mn	Manganese	.123500
Au	Gold	.000006	Mo	Molybdenum	.001592
B	Boron	.019400	N	Nitrogen	1.467000
Ba	Barium	.001276	Na	Sodium	4.180000
Be	Beryllium	Trace	Ni	Nickel	.003500
Bi	Bismuth	Trace	O	Oxygen	Undeclared
Br	Bromine	Trace	Os	Osmium	Trace
C	Carbon	Undeclared	P	Phosphorus	.211000
Ca	Calcium	1.904000	Pb	Lead	.000014
Cb	Niobium	Trace	Pd	Palladium	Trace
Cd	Cadmium	Trace	Pl	Platinum	Trace
Ce	Cerium	Trace	Ra	Radium	Trace
Cl	Chlorine	3.680000	Rb	Rubidium	.000005
Co	Cobalt	.001227	Rh	Rhodium	Trace
Cr	Chromium	Trace	S	Sulphur	1.564200
Cs	Caesium	Trace	Se	Selenium	.000043
Cu	Copper	.000635	Sb	Antimony	.000142
F	Fluorine	.032650	Si	Silicon	.164200
Fe	Iron	.089560	Sn	Tin	.000006
Ga	Gallium	Trace	Sr	Strontium	.074876
Ge	Germanium	.000006	Te	Tellurium	Trace
H	Hydrogen	Undeclared	Th	Thorium	Trace
Hg	Mercury	.000190	Ti	Titanium	.000012
I	Iodine	.062400	Tl	Thallium	.000293
Id	Indium	Trace	U	Uranium	.000004
Ir	Irridium	Trace	V	Vanadium	.000531
K	Potassium	1.280000	W	Tungsten	.000033
La	Lantanum	.000019	Zn	Zinc	.003516
Li	Lithium	.000007	Zr	Zirconium	Trace

seaweeds. I believe Dr. Kondo's conclusions are correct and that his study is one from which we can learn how to live a long life. Now the Japanese have become a people with the longest lifespan in the world, the Japanese woman's average lifespan being almost eighty years. Fifty years ago it was only forty-five years; although this increase is mainly due to decreased infant death, it is still amazing.

Fruits

Many people say "fruits and vegetables" in the same breath, but actually they are much different. There is no doubt that vegetables are more valuable than fruits in terms of nutrients for our body. Many people believe that fruit was the principal food of our ancestors, but I don't think this is true. Fruits have special ripening seasons and cannot provide a stable food supply. Also, they cannot be stored. Leaves, roots, nuts, and seeds were undoubtedly eaten more frequently.

Around the middle of the nineteenth century one of the great teachers in the health field, Sylvester Graham, was advocating fruits as food. Despite his many excellent ideas, he did not live long; in 1851 he died at the age of fifty-six. Until Graham's time fruits were considered to be a dangerous food among both Europeans and Americans. It is interesting to guess how this trend began. The tuberculosis epidemic, a disease thought to be incurable, had its peak at this time. For about two hundred years tuberculosis had been prevalent in Europe, and both the cause and the treatment were as yet unknown. But people discovered just through observation and experience that the incidences of the disease were related to the high consumption of fruit. About this same time sugar was being imported from the East and, while sugar was in fact a more powerful co-factor in the development of the disease, people were unaware of the connection, as they are to this day. But they did think there was some relation between fruit and the disease.

From the end of the eighteenth century into the nineteenth, agricultural techniques underwent a remarkable development. People began eating a lot of meat and therefore needed to eat more carbohydrates. As we have seen, raw vegetables, fresh fruits, large amounts of potatoes, and a low-salt diet are all related to heavy meat consumption.

My opinion on fruits is neutral – I do not say they are good or bad. Fruit with meat, eggs, or other animal products is a good combination. Fruit with sugar is not. From a nutritional standpoint the reason for this is clear. While meat contains large amounts of protein and fat, it is lacking in carbohydrates, minerals, and some vitamins. Fruits, on the other hand, contain lots of carbohydrates, minerals, various vitamins, but are short on protein and fat. Most people whose diets consist of a variety of foods can eat fruit on occasion without any problem.

Why do people enjoy eating fruits? The special character of fruits is their sweetness. Usually fruits contain about 10 to 40 percent sugar, mainly as fructose, the simplest form of carbohydrate. This means that the sugar passes quickly into the bloodstream from the digestive tract, thus satisfying busy people's desire for a quick balance with high protein in the blood, but with similar, unfavorable effects as common sugar.

Generally, fruits are high in potassium, an important nutrient, but either lack salt or are low in sodium and chlorine. Our potassium/sodium balance should always be maintained. Potassium chloride and sodium chloride work together in practically all parts of our bodies. The body cells are rich in potassium, and in the blood sodium dominates (see Table 5). However, through daily excretions such as the urine, we lose more sodium than potassium (see Table 6). We lose even more salt through sweat, mucus, tears, and other fluids. Thus it is good to add salt to our cooking, especially with a vegetarian diet. Too much potassium or sodium can create a malfunction of the nervous system; excess potassium will cause numbness, muscle spasms, and paralysis, whereas too much sodium will tend to make our nerves hypersensitive and restless. The heart is always working in a cycle of contraction and expansion. Potassium accounts for the expansion, sodium for the contraction. They always work together as a team. If the sodium level in the blood

Table 5. Electrolyte Composition of Body Fluids

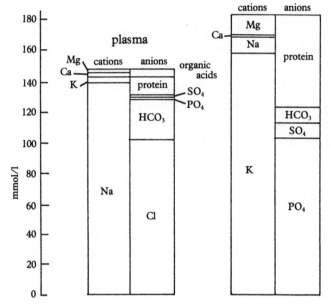

Table 6. Relative Composition of Plasma and Urine in Normal Men[4]

	Plasma g/100 ml	Urine g/100 ml	Concentration in urine
Water	90-93	95	–
Proteins and other colloids	7-8.5	–	–
Urea	0.03	2	x 60
Uric acid	0.002	0.03	x 15
Glucose	0.1	–	–
Creatinine	0.001	0.1	x 100
Sodium	0.32	0.6	x 2
Potassium	0.02	0.15	x 7
Calcium	0.01	0.015	x 1.5
Magnesium	0.0025	0.01	x 4
Chloride	0.37	0.6	x 2
Phosphate	0.003	0.12	x 40
Sulfate	0.003	0.18	x 60
Ammonia	0.0001	0.05	x 500

decreases, the heart loses its power to contract, thereby failing in its work of moving the blood through the body.

As a rule people don't overeat vegetables, since their flavors are simple and their comparatively greater volume and bulk quickly fills our stomachs. Fruits, on the other hand, are sweet and easily eaten to excess. I have known of people who were capable of eating ten pounds of watermelon in one sitting. This is clearly overeating.

In this country one group refers to themselves as fruitarians, claiming to eat fruit almost exclusively. Some of them take no salt. Most likely this is a reaction to heavy meat-eating in the past. However, they can't stay healthy very long this way. It is difficult for fruitarians to get sufficient protein, fat, and salt in their diet. If they eat some eggs or other animal foods, their preference for fruit would be more understandable.

The best way to eat fruit is from tree to mouth. Eat them raw, ripe, and with the skin whenever possible. Plant strawberries and watermelons in your garden and eat them there. You can enjoy delicious, perfect fruits. Commercial fruit, on the other hand, is picked before it is ripe in order to send it to faraway places where it is stored for many days; it is less tasty, harder to digest, and often contains strong acids which can cause decalcification in the body. Some children have been killed by eating prematured fruits which contain a form of cyanide.

As for dried or cooked fruits, this is not the best way to eat them; it is best to eat a limited amount, diluted by water and with other foods, as dry fruits especially are very sweet and concentrated. Their character is closer to common sugar (see Table 8). These fruits contain calcium, but not enough to balance such high sugar content.

Today, many kinds of fruit are available almost everywhere, whenever you want them. But these are also not the best quality; fruit should be eaten in season and in its own locality. In the summer we have plums, apricots, prunes, peaches, and then watermelon; in the fall, pears and apples; in the winter, tangerines

Table 7. Nutritional Content of Vegetables and Fruits[5]

		Vegetables				Fruits				Dried Fruit
		Cabbage	Carrot	Lettuce	Onion	Apple	Grape	Orange	Water-melon	Raisins
Water	%	92.4	88.2	94.0	89.1	84.4	81.6	86.0	92.6	18.0
Protein	g	1.3	1.1	1.3	1.5	0.2	1.3	1.0	0.5	2.5
Fat	g	0.2	0.2	0.3	0.1	0.6	1.0	0.2	0.2	0.2
Carbohydrate	g	5.4	9.7	3.5	3.7	14.5	15.7	12.2	6.4	77.4
Fiber	g	0.8	1.0	0.7	0.6	1.0	0.6	0.5	0.3	0.9
Ash	g	0.7	0.8	0.9	0.6	0.3	0.4	0.6	0.3	1.9
Calcium	mg	49.0	37.0	68.0	27.0	7.0	16.0	41.0	7.0	62.0
Phosphorus	mg	29.0	36.0	25.0	36.0	10.0	12.0	20.0	10.0	101.0
Iron	mg	0.4	0.7	1.4	0.5	0.3	0.4	0.4	0.5	3.5
Sodium	mg	20.0	47.0	9.0	10.0	1.0	3.0	1.0	1.0	27.0
Potassium	mg	233.0	341.0	264.0	157.0	110.0	158.0	194.0	100.0	763.0
Vitamin A	I.N.	130.0	11,000.0	1,900.0	40.0	90.0	100.0	260.0	590.0	20.0
Thiamine B_1	mg	0.05	0.06	9.06	9.03	0.03	0.05	0.1	0.03	0.11
Riboflavin B_2	mg	0.05	0.05	0.06	0.04	0.02	0.03	0.04	0.03	0.03
Niacin B_3	mg	0.3	0.6	0.3	0.2	0.1	0.3	0.4	0.2	0.5
Ascorbic Acid	mg	47.0	8.0	6.0	10.0	4.0	4.0	50.0	7.0	1.0

	Bananas	Dates	Figs	Plums	Grapes	Raisins	Apples	Apricots
Fresh	22.2	–	20.3	16.6	15.7	–	14.5	12.8
Dried	88.6	72.9	69.1	67.4	–	77.4	71.8	68.3

Table 8. Percent Carbohydrate in Fresh and Dried Fruits[6]

followed by grapefruit; in the spring, strawberries and then cherries. So we see that in this country plenty of fruits are naturally available all year round. We have no reason to buy imported fruit. In the tropics, the sun's energy and the special environment create a different quality of food. Tropical foods are suitable for tropical people. Imported fruits are all sterilized by means of strong chemicals intended not only to protect the plants and fruits from disease, but also to counteract various dangerous diseases which exist only in the tropics. Still, it would be difficult to say that such fruits are safe to eat, especially bananas that have been ripened by gas, for example.

Vegetarianism

We cannot talk about vegetables without talking about vegetarians. To be a vegetarian means eating plant foods only, not vegetables only. Today many people are changing their diets for a variety of reasons. The United States Department of Agriculture (USDA) estimates that at least 5 percent of the United States population is predominantly vegetarian, but even this small percentage represents more than ten million people and is growing daily. Medical and scientific evidence indicates that, statistically, vegetarians in the United States are thinner, healthier, and may live longer than meat-eaters.

People turn away from meat for a variety of reasons. The majority of the world's population seldom eats meat, more out of necessity than by choice, since meat is usually the most expensive of foods. In the Far East, religious teachings and spiritual practices have traditionally favored a vegetarian diet and in the West there are also several religious and monastic orders that practice vegetarian or near-vegetarian diets.

A minority of vegetarians are against the killing of animals for clothing or for food. Many present-day vegetarians have chosen a no-meat or low-meat diet because of environmental and health concerns. Some feel that a vegetarian diet makes the most sense for the most people, so vegetarianism can be seen as one way of understanding the ecological limitations of a crowded planet. Complete vegetarians, or vegans, eat no meat or animal-related foods. Lacto-vegetarians will drink milk and eat yogurt and cheese. The lacto-ovo-vegetarians add eggs to their dairy intake. (Eating eggs is not seen as killing, since non-fertile eggs are devoid of life.) Pesco-vegetarians permit themselves some fish.

The number of people who follow a strict vegan diet is not exactly known, but probably there are not so many. Strict vegetarians may not live so long, since vegetables alone, with their low protein and fat, are not a balanced diet. While beans, seeds, and nuts along with grain can provide a diet rich in protein and fats, I recommend an occasional amount of protein from some animal source. If not, a very large quantity of foods must be eaten to provide sufficient amounts of certain nutrients.

In extremely destitute countries where many cannot ever eat animal food, people have been known to eat as much as five pounds of food at one sitting; over time, this can only result in digestive and other troubles. Long-lived people around the world have shown us that a strictly vegetarian diet is not the best; small amounts of animal food are eaten on occasion. In Asian countries many famous Buddhist priests who followed strict vegan diets did not live so long, maybe only to fifty or fifty-five; compared to others – artists, writers, politicians – it is hard to say they had long lives. Table 9 shows the lifespans of some famous vegetarians.

Many vegetarians have had long lives, but ironically the great dramatist of irony, Bernard Shaw, had the longest life of all. He was a very strong advocate of vegetarianism and called himself a

Table 9. Famous Vegetarians

				Age
Philosophers	Pythagoras	B.C.	580-500?	80
and Religious	Buddha		563-481?	82
Teachers	Socrates		470-399	70 (suicide)
	Plato		428-347	80
	Seneca	A.D.	54-139	84
	St. Francis		1182-1226	43
	Voltaire		1694-1778	83
	Dalai Lama		1391-1475	83
	Dogen		1200-1253	52
	Mahatma Gandhi		1867-1948	79 (killed)
Scientists	Isaac Newton		1643-1727	83
	Charles Darwin		1809-1882	72
	Albert Einstein		1879-1955	75
	Albert Schweitzer		1875-1965	89
Writers	Plutarch		46-120?	74
	John Milton		1608-1674	65
	Jean Jacques Rousseau		1712-1778	65
	Ralph Waldo Emerson		1803-1882	78
	Henry David Thoreau		1817-1863	45
	Rabindranath Tagore		1817-1905	87
	Leo Tolstoy		1878-1910	81
	George Bernard Shaw		1856-1950	93
	Upton Sinclair		1878-1968	89
	H. B. Wells		1866-1946	79
	Leonardo Da Vinci		1452-1519	66

vegetarian, but actually he would eat anything on occasion. It is estimated that his diet consisted of more than 99 percent plant food, so his deviation of 0.3 or 0.5 percent was negligible in comparison with other people. We can therefore still refer to him as a vegetarian, and this is probably the best way for a long life.

Another example is Dogen, a famous Buddhist who founded one of the Zen schools in Japan about eight hundred years ago. Now that Dogen's writings are being translated and are reaching the

Western world, his name is being ranked among the great philosophers of history. Born to a noble family, Dogen could likely have eaten anything he wanted when he was young. At the age of twelve he became a monk. From then on he ate a purely vegetarian diet, but unfortunately he died at the age of fifty-three. Shinran, a contemporary of Dogen, was also from a noble family. At the age of eight he, too, became a monk. But in his late twenties he broke the admonition of the teaching that had come down from Gautama Buddha prohibiting the eating of meat. Shinran ate some fish and also married. He was courageous and honest and was responsible for a reform of Japanese Buddhism, comparable to the changes brought about by Martin Luther in the Christian church about three hundred years later. Shinran lived until the age of eighty-three.

If we compare the lives of these two philosophers, we could say that Dogen's life work was completed in about twenty years while Shinran's lasted more than fifty. Both left many books we can read now. It appears that Dogen's spiritual development may have exceeded Shinran's, and he had a great influence on Japanese culture. Whether Dogen was a genius or whether his greatness resulted from his strict vegetarian diet is difficult to say. It is possible to have a genius who eats sugar and fruit, such as British poet Percy Bysshe Shelley (1792-1822), who lived only thirty years and died of tuberculosis. We can see that vegetarianism and sugar-eating is a catastrophic combination.

I was a pure vegetarian for more than six years. I consumed about two pounds of brown rice daily, but I was always hungry. After considering many examples in the history of human food and reflecting on our ancestors' evolutionary process, I decided to give up being a pure vegetarian and began to eat small amounts of animal food. Today I am about 99.8 percent vegetarian. Still, I feel guilty for eating animal food. I don't fish or hunt, but I do buy these foods; this means I am ordering fishermen or butchers to kill animals.

Milk

It seems that the Buddha was a lacto-vegetarian, although not much is written about his eating habits. However, his most important recommendation was, "Don't kill anything." One clearly written story about him is that he tried to follow the practice of fasting as recommended by the Brahmans. After many days, he gave up trying to be a Brahman and drank some cow's milk brought to him by a young girl. He recovered from the exhaustion of fasting. He then began Zen meditation and reached enlightenment.

The Russian physiologist Elie Metchnikoff did extensive research on the long-lived peoples of the Caucasus mountains. He concluded that their long life was attributable mainly to their eating yogurt. He stressed that fermented foods are favorable for longevity. About this same time Rudolf Steiner began teaching the lacto-vegetarian diet. He said that for our spiritual development we should be vegetarians but that milk is the human's most basic food, provided it was consumed raw and unpasteurized.

I don't agree that cow's or goat's milk are the best foods for human beings, but they were probably the best protein source until the early part of the twentieth century. Since that time the more developed chemical industries have been creating pollution in the air, the water, and the soil everywhere. Large amounts of fertilizers, insecticides, herbicides, and other chemicals are sprayed over the farmlands where the herds are grazed; the animals eat contaminated plants, and these contaminants are probably more concentrated in their milk and in their meat, especially in their livers.

The latest discovery is a special hormone capable of stimulating the production of cow's milk to double the amount. This seems to be a great discovery, but it is too good to believe and it is likely that something is wrong with the quality of milk thus produced. Chemical analyses of this milk have not yet been reported. Even if chemical analysis were to show no difference in quality from milk produced without hormones, people know by taste and stomach that something is wrong, for the consumption of milk and other dairy products is decreasing rapidly. Milk is no longer a good food. And if the milk is bad, then cheese, butter, yogurt and all the products made from that milk are the same. For these reasons, I don't recommend dairy products as a part of your daily diet.

Chapter 8

Salt

Crystal of The Sea

Salt and water, like sunshine and air, are more than food; they are the essence of life. Ever since primitive life first emerged in the ancient oceans animal cells have always lived in a bath of sea water. Scientists speculate that at least 3.5 billion years ago life began in the warm ocean with the appearance of tiny, microscopic, single-celled living organisms. The sea water was their blood, bringing them nutrients and oxygen and carrying their waste products away. Slowly these single-celled organisms evolved into more complex, multi-celled organisms, but always the sea water was their blood. Once they became complex enough that some of their cells were not exposed to the sea-blood outside, they had to circulate it inside themselves to provide the same life-giving nutrients and functions. This eventually allowed living creatures to leave the ocean, but to carry some of this saline solution inside, pumped and circulated around to bathe each cell as had been done for the first forms of life.

Now we have the magnificent human being, looking much different from that first single-celled ancestor, yet if we look at our individual cells, we find that they are still living in the same way. Our body fluids are essentially of the same composition as that ancient sea water, all of our 75 trillion body cells receiving nutrients and oxygen and excreting waste products in the very same ways: We can witness the entire evolution of life on earth by noticing what happens when egg and sperm meet in a saline solution and combine to begin new life. At this moment our body again goes back to the one-celled organism and begins to grow, bathed in the sea water called the amniotic fluid. The fetus at times resembles a worm, then a fish, and next a reptile and then a rodent (see p. 170).

At the time our ancestors left the sea with the salty liquid now enclosed within, the sea water was far less concentrated than it is at present. That is the reason our blood and body fluids are not as salty as the ocean is now. Even the blood of ocean fish is not so salty, and the bodies of other sea animals also are not salty. But still there is salt and water in all our body fluids – blood, lymph, mucus, urine, sweat, tears, saliva, and so on. We always lose salt when we urinate and sweat, so it is necessary to replace it by taking a little salt every day.

Once our ancestors left the ocean, they would return to the sea if they needed salt and take in salty marsh weeds, sea weeds, or sea water. Long before humans developed agriculture, our ancestors were eating salt. This has been shown by new archeological studies of charred food remains at ancient camp sites.

Salt, Wealth, Power, and Civilization

Human civilizations were supported through the cultivation of food; as populations grew, more food was needed. Salt was especially important, and therefore the first civilization appeared in the area of Sodom, located in the region where salt was produced naturally. This was about eight or nine thousand years ago. In ancient China, too, people settled near the mouth of the Yellow River, and this is still the major salt-producing area in China today.

Not only humans but almost all animals need salt, especially herbivorous animals, which often search out and visit salt deposits over great distances and with the same determination with which they seek out water. Everyone knows that cows and horses need salt, and wild animals often take salt from the urine of other animals. If bee keepers don't feed salt to the honeybees, they will also take it from animal urine. Monkeys were thought to be an exception to this need, but this was wrong. Monkeys are always eating lice and fleas or salt crystals from their sweat. Since salt is the most important component of blood, all animals take salt.

Many wars were fought and empires built over the need for salt, and for the lack of it these same empires collapsed. In ancient Rome a special road was built for transporting salt to the city; it was called the Via Salaria. Troops of soldiers protected and carried the salt, and the money they received for their labor was called salarium (salary). Historically, the price of salt has often been as high or higher than the price of gold; one pound of salt might have been worth about $5,000 in today's money.

Salt played an important role in history and the development of human culture. Around 500 A.D. the Mediterranean and Atlantic sea levels rose about six feet, covering the salt beds. The Romans and many Europeans lost power and the Dark Ages descended upon Europe. At the same time the Arab countries flourished, maintaining their power through the trading of salt. By about the tenth century the seas subsided and the salt beds were once more accessible. People again began producing and using salt, the Dark Ages gradually faded out, and the great European Renaissance began. This period also marked the beginning of the Crusades. All these events are more than mere coincidence.

Historians say that if the French soldiers had had enough salt when Napoleon invaded Russia, they would not have lost so many men.

American independence was once threatened by Lord Howe's attempt to gain control over salt supplies; many battles were fought over salt. During the Civil War, too, the North occupied all the sources of salt and blocked the South from importing it.

At some points in history salt became so expensive that people were known to have traded their lives for it, becoming slaves for salt. There are records of American slave traders buying children in Africa for a handful of salt.

To control the Asian people, the British government imposed strict taxes over all the salt trading in India. Mahatma Gandhi succeeded in breaking this system without using violence.

Divine Food

Everywhere we look we see the importance of salt. Homer, the ancient Greek poet, wrote, "Salt is divine." Plato hailed salt as "Dear to the gods." In the New Testament, Jesus says: "Salt is good; but if the salt has lost its saltness, how will you season it? Have salt in yourselves; and be at peace with one another." (Mark 9:50) And again, in Matthew: "You are the salt of the earth . . ." (5:13) In many cultures, salt was and is a holy food that is served to God or spirit.

It was not only a food, but was also considered a medicine by many peoples. Again we see that salt is practically synonymous with life; it is the positive, dynamic factor that protects and animates the body of mankind and the life of the spirit as well.

In 1974, a Japanese soldier, Lt. Hiroo Onoda, returned from a small island in the Phillipines after thirty years of hiding in the jungle since the beginning of World War II. During a meeting with journalists, someone asked him, "What gave you the most suffering?" He replied without hesitation, "The shortage of salt."

Meat-eating and Salt

At the beginning of the nineteenth century Friedrich Christian Oetinger wrote the following: "Salt is a marvellous thing; it is possessed of the loftiest and most glorious nature, and is God's greatest, sublimest work in the whole realm of nature. There is nothing material that can compare with it. It is a subject and a mystery never yet penetrated, and never to be fully penetrated."[1]

This is a wonderful statement, but why was it necessary to

emphasize the importance of salt, long known by common sense? Less than twenty years earlier, in 1789, the monopoly held by the French monarchy over salt and its high price led to the French Revolution; in establishing the free trading of salt, the people also acquired power and equal rights from the royal family and the nobility. This revolutionary time of the late eighteenth century, the age of the bourgeoisie, began with the issue of people's basic right to salt.

So precious and valued was the crystal of the sea that the famous Italian artist Benvenuto Cellini made a salt container of gold, enamel, and ebony for the French king. This piece is now in the collection of the Winna Museum in Austria.

As a result of industry's development, improved agricultural technology, and increased commodity trading, the middle class people of the late eighteenth century quickly became rich and began to eat a lot of meat as the royal families and nobles had done before. This decreased the importance of salt. Meat was the most expensive food, not affordable by the poor. The foods of the ancient Romans were so luxurious that they often referred to gout as the "royal disease."

By the middle of the nineteenth century, hundreds of thousands of people in Europe had gout, encouraging strong reactions against the intake of salty foods. Benjamin Franklin said that meat should be eaten sparingly. (Today gout is causing pain and discomfort for more than 1.8 million Americans from all walks of life.[2]) It was after this time that William Metcalf, Sylvester Graham, and other famous vegetarian teachers appeared. In 1847 the British Vegetarian Society was established. As heavy meat-eating increased, so did interest in vegetarianism.

Organic and Inorganic Minerals

Justus von Liebig (1803-1873), one of the most influential chemists of the nineteenth century, researched biochemistry and agricultural chemistry and taught that minerals should be taken only in organic form. This is almost right, but is not perfect. To realize this, the only thing one can do is to drink animal's blood, but these days no one practices such a thing. At that time the scientific world was divided by two opposing ideas on salt. Some said that the mineral form of salt was not necessary; others considered it essential for life.

We have seen that salt and water are the fundamental substances of our blood, as they are in the ocean. Here is an example that illustrates their importance. In 1882 a British doctor, Sidney Ringer, found that body tissue cells (in his first experiments, a frog's heart) could stay alive in a salt solution. If he put them into plain water, they would absorb too much of it, swell up, and explode. The following solution of certain minerals was found to keep body cells alive for a long time:

0.87 gram of sodium chloride (NaCl)
0.02 gram of potassium chloride (KCl)
0.03 gram of calcium chloride ($CaCl_2$)

This became the prototype for a blood substitute used in blood transfusions known as the Ringer Solution, which has saved many lives. He also tested 0.05 gram of potassium chloride instead of 0.02 gram and found that the cells died very quickly. Cells are that sensitive.

Another researcher, Rene Kenton, studied the similarity of sea water and human and animal blood and was able to show that our ancestors came from the sea.

If all our body cells need to be bathed in this salty mineral water solution in order to stay alive and function, then we can understand that once the blood runs low on salt, the cells may stop working properly and can die. The average human body has about seven ounces (almost half a pound) of salt and the blood is maintaining a similar proportion. We must pay special attention to the fact that in our blood there is salt, not merely sodium and chlorine, and that the body will separate out and utilize the elements as it requires.

Salt-Restricted Vegetarian Diet

The first person in the scientific world to question and clearly recommend a limit on salt consumption was probably Bircher-Benner, a German physician successful in following a vegetarian diet. At that time (toward the end of the nineteenth century), salt consumption in civilized countries was estimated to have been twenty to thirty grams per day. Bircher-Benner determined that the daily intake of salt should not exceed three to five grams.[3]

Gustav V. Bunge (1844-1920) carefully studied salt consumption and summarized his findings as follows:

1. Sodium chloride is necessary in mineral form.
2. The requirement for sodium chloride is higher when the diet consists primarily of plant foods.
3. The requirement for sodium chloride is lower when the diet consists primarily of meat and animal foods; in fact, too much salt can be taken in.
4. Sodium chloride and potassium interact within the organism. Plant foods contain three to four times more potassium than meat. The wealth of potassium in plants causes an increased salt requirement for those who eat a primarily vegetarian diet.[4]

This is a beautiful and fair summary. But in spite of Bunge's work, meat-eating continued to increase markedly. Discussion on salt consumption has continued to the present day. In the United States the majority of scientists and physicians are nearly agreed on the negative side, and now salt is something like the new villain or poison of our times. In recent years I have seen no writings on the necessity of mineral salt in our diet (aside from the recommendations of *Dietary Goals for the United States,* pp. 49-51).

If a more vegetarian diet is recommended, then more salt also is needed. Another possible reason for the loss of interest in salt is the change in its quality and taste.

The Quality of Salt

Contrary to what we have been led to believe, salt is not just sodium chloride. Good quality salt must include all the various minerals that are found in sea water – this is what I mean when I say salt.

Within the last hundred years or so the quality of salt has changed completely. The salt now available in stores is all refined salt. Some labels read "99.999% sodium chloride." It stings the tongue and throat when eaten, and looks like a chemical drug. For millions of years our ancestors never ate such purified salt; only modern man has broken the millions-of-years-old biological tradition of having true unrefined sea salt in the blood. Calcium and iodine are added to this refined "salt" to provide some essential mineral nutrition, and dextrose to moderate the sharp taste. In addition, a substance to prevent caking is added to some salt, which actually prevents it from combining with water. This salt is useless to the body; instead of being a vital food, it has been reduced to a flavoring agent.

What probably contributed to this misunderstanding about salt was the scientific discovery that the salty taste our tongue recognizes comes from the chemical compound sodium chloride (NaCl). Many people incorrectly understood this to mean that sodium chloride must be salt. NaCl is not salt. Ironically, new research has found that potassium chloride has almost the same taste as sodium chloride, even though it has existed in sea water in small amounts for billions of years prior to this discovery, and it is available today as a salt substitute. However, large amounts of this salt are quite toxic.

Pure Salt is Mineral Deficient

Generally, American salt companies are manufacturing 99.7 percent pure sodium chloride and calling it salt, based on a 1913 ruling requiring that salt used for human consumption must be more than 99 percent sodium chloride. This is a strange law to impose in the home of liberty. I believe that the passage of this law coincided with the time when Americans began losing their vitality.

A clear sign of this change was a decline in the birth rate. The relationship between salt and infertility was seen in the early 1900s by American ranchers when their cows were not reproducing. Researchers found that certain minerals missing in the salt was the cause. Once these minerals were added to the salt licks, the cows again began producing plenty of calves. All the salt made for animal feed now includes the additional necessary minerals. We know that deficiencies of certain minerals can cause both sterility and infertility in humans as well as animals. But the problem is not limited to the birth rate; both physical endurance and the American pioneer spirit seem to have been reduced.

We must understand our need for good quality salt with all its minerals and obtain it with the same natural determination as the animals.

Salt and Water Balance

The study of human blood is very complicated. Red blood globules are made to carry oxygen more efficiently and many kinds of white blood cells and other defense materials are produced to fight against pathogens. There are platelets and other substances to stop bleeding. The blood also carries warmness and coolness to keep the body at an optimal temperature, prevent the overheating of the internal organs, and keep the extremities warm. The endocrine glands produce more than a hundred hormones to control bodily functions. Everything rides on this great transportation system of blood. But still the basic materials of blood are salt and water.

Maintaining the right proportion and amount of salt and water is crucially important for life and good health. Many organs work together for this purpose: kidneys; adrenal glands; skin; intestines; saliva glands; pituitary glands; and finally the supreme commander, the brain. All information and instructions are carried to and from the brain by the nervous system and by hormonal secretions. For example, if the body has an excess of water, the kidneys excrete more water and reabsorb more salt. The intestines absorb less water and the skin excretes more sweat. If the body loses water by perspiration or for any other reason, the kidneys excrete more salt and reabsorb more water, less water evaporates from the skin and the body feels thirsty. Less saliva is produced and the mouth and throat dry up. We drink water and the thirst is stopped immediately before the small intestines absorb the water. If the body loses salt and water in extremely hot weather or by sitting in a hot room, high fever, vomiting, diarrhea, or other disorders associated with dehydration can occur. Even if enough water is supplied, the kidneys cannot hold it without salt. Death can result. Make sure to take enough salt and water.

But before such a serious condition arises, the normal body feels thirsty and one drinks water. And if one feels low energy, weakness of muscles, or no will power to continue working, the body will want some salty food.

How Much Salt to Take

Scientists are trying to determine how much salt we need and how much we are consuming. This is a difficult problem. Some people drink a lot of beer or soft drinks and others drink very little. Meat eaters and vegetarians are different. Some people actively produce much sweat and others don't. Also, many commercial foods contain salt. Actually, I have never seen anyone checking foods exactly with a gram or milligram scale. Approximate amounts of salt can be calculated in schools and hospitals, but many questions remain. How much of each dish did each person eat? How much was left over? Were salty condiments added at the table? It is hard to check one by one.

The estimate is that Americans consume about twenty grams of salt per day per person, Asians take about thirty grams a day. More than fourteen grams of salt per day is considered an excess, but as long as many Americans are drinking large amounts of soft drinks, coffee, and other liquids, this amount seems reasonable. It would be better to reduce both liquid and salt intake. Since most people have no food analysis charts and no scale, when anyone recommends a salt reduction, some people begin a no-salt diet. Eating no salt can be more dangerous; you have to watch your needs carefully.

Actually, people are taking salt by intuition and not many mistakes are made except among people who have taken both salt and meat. Even children don't make mistakes. For newborn babies, an adequate amount of salt comes from mother's milk; they will spit out a salt solution if it is given. I think millions of years of tradition and habit went into the gene's memory. It is very uncomfortable to take an excessive amount of salt.

When you go to a restaurant the salt shaker is always sitting in the center of the table. Have you ever thought why? This is telling you, "We did our best in preparing this food for you, but we don't know exactly how much salt you need. Please determine this for yourself."

Still, great care should be taken. The best way to determine the right amount is to chew your food very well to try to achieve the best taste possible with minor adjustments of salt. The food should not taste salty or too mild. If you chew well, your tongue can determine this for you.

Other Functions of Salt (Sodium)

In solution, sodium and chlorine separate and some of these atoms, called ions, carry an electrical charge. Sodium carries a positive electrical charge (Na+) and makes the body more alkaline, and chlorine carries a negative charge (Cl-) which creates acid. Potassium (+), phosphorus (-), and other elements also make ions and are called electrolytes.

Actually, sodium and potassium ions regulate the water balance in the body. They also have an important role as nerve transmitters, and make the muscles contract and expand, including the heart muscle. Another function of sodium is to keep other blood minerals soluble so they will not build up as deposits in the bloodstream. It acts with chlorine to improve blood and lymph health, and helps purge carbon dioxide from the body. Through salt deficiency our nerve cells can lose their function, bringing about numbness, muscle cramps, weight loss, reduced growth, nausea, diarrhea, and headache. In digestion, salt creates a good appetite by stimulating the taste buds and salivary glands.

Functions of Chlorine

Chlorine, a strong-smelling, greenish-yellow gas, never exists in nature as a single element, but its compounds, such as sodium chloride, are widespread. All kinds of chlorine compounds are toxic with the one exception of salt.

The body contains about one hundred grams (four ounces) of chlorine, which represents about 0.15 percent of an average person's weight, most of which is combined with sodium or potassium. It is found mainly in the blood and lymph fluid, but it is present in red blood cells and the cells of other tissues. The blood contains 0.51 percent chlorine, 0.34 percent sodium, and 0.02 to 0.22 percent potassium; thus the chlorine content of blood is higher than any other mineral.[5] The highest concentration of body chlorine is found in the gastric juice and in the cerebral-spinal fluid.

The chloride ion, which is negatively charged, plays a major role in the regulation of osmotic pressure, water balance, and acid-alkaline balance. It is also required by the stomach for the production of hydrochloric acid. This acid is necessary for the digestion of protein; it also absorbs vitamin B_{12} and iron, suppressing the growth of microorganisms which enter the stomach with food and drink.

During the past two hundred years there has been no shortage of salt in developed countries, and so no chlorine deficiencies have ever been reported there. But in recent years injudicious use of diuretic drugs, or strict vegetarian diets applied without salt, have resulted in severe chlorine deficiencies leading to alkalosis, a condition characterized by slow and shallow breathing, listlessness, muscle cramps, lack of appetite, and occasionally convulsions.

Some researchers say that chlorine stimulates the liver to function as a filter for wastes and helps to clear toxic waste products out of the system. It also aids in keeping joints and tendons in youthful shape and in the distribution of hormones through the body.[6]

Chlorine is often added to water for purification purposes as it destroys water-borne disease such as typhoid and dysentery. There is some question as to whether added chlorine in the water is also toxic for the human body, since it is a highly reactive chemical and may join with other chemicals to form harmful substances. It is known that chlorine in drinking water destroys vitamin E and also kills intestinal bacteria helpful in the digestion of food.

We can say that salt is a strange material from its birth. Sodium (Na) is a metal which bursts into flame when exposed to water. Chlorine (Cl) is a gas. Each is a lethal poison, but when combined, they fuse with each other completely and become a life-sustaining material, salt. Our body is a magician, the way it can separate these poisons and recombine them to make hydrochloric acid and other substances. The chemical industry utilizes this double character; fertilizer made from salt can produce green fields and rich crops, but insecticides can be made from the same chemical. Salt can also be made into herbicides which kill plants that many animals need for their survival.

Between birth and death is our life. Salt gives us life, but Death Valley is a valley of salt deposits. In the Dead Sea no fish are living. Salt is a strong preservative, meaning it can kill bacteria and fungi, or at least inhibit their growth and activity. Chlorine is especially effective for killing living organisms. According to botanical research, the only mineral not essential for plant growth is chlorine; plants can grow in soil with or without chlorine. If chlorine combines with sodium, it is stable and safe to eat, but if it combines with other elements, it can turn suddenly to poison. Even potassium chloride is not safe to take in large amounts. If we calculate the daily chlorine loss from urination, we find that nine grams a day

Table 9. Urine Constituents[7]
(g/24 hours)

Urea	25-30
Uric acid	0.6-0.7
Creatinine	1.0-1.2
Hippuric acid	0.7
Ammonia	0.7
Amino acids	3.0
Sodium	1-5 (NaCl 15.0)
Potassium	2-4
Calcium	0.2-0.3
Magnesium	0.1
Chloride	7.0
Phosphate	1.7-2.5
Sulfate	1.8-2.5
Iron	0.003

are lost in six cups of urine; fifteen grams in ten cups.

Sea Minerals and Obesity

You may laugh, but the following is a true story. For a long time, at least one thousand years, the Japanese respected and envied fat people. For they were a slim people, and fat persons were seldom to be seen. The illustrations shown here are examples.

Figure 6. Ebisu and Daikoku

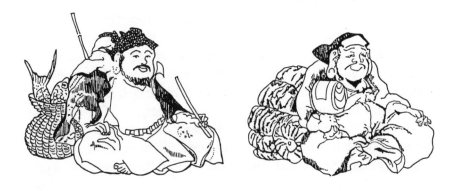

These two popular figures, Ebisu and Daikoku, were the symbol of wealth and happiness. Many people tried but failed to have such a body. Surely this story sounds like a dream.

From a nutritional standpoint, overweight is caused just by excess calories. If we take in more calories than we use, we gain weight. But the question remains, why couldn't the Japanese become obese? People who overeat are found in all cultures. Then, after World War II, an incredible thing happened. Young Japanese children began gaining weight. Now almost the entire population has gotten fatter, and still the Japanese are optimistic because a big body is desirable and looks healthier. For a thousand years their ancestors wanted such a body. To me this is very strange. I have thought about this for a long time and I know that a fat body is not healthier; generally, fat people are weaker against infections, and some researchers say that white blood cell activity is slowed down in an overweight body, which is even more serious. But the changes in foods or diet among the Japanese have been relatively small. They had already learned to eat meat and drink milk a hundred years before, and sugar and bread were introduced about three hundred years ago; these have slowly become popular in Japan.

The only new factor I can connect to this increase in obesity is the quality of salt. Before World War II the Japanese were using refined salt only in salt shakers on the dining table. But following the war the cooking salt used in the kitchen, as well as that used by food industries, has all been refined salt. They had lost something in the salt. In Japan there are still some groups of people resisting the use of refined salt by using special salt made by traditional methods. (Among these groups of people there are almost no fat people.) Scientists have identified about seventy-five kinds of elements in sea water, but theoretically there could be ninety-two, all of the earth materials. Probably we need all these trace elements, but around thirty have been determined as essential minerals needed on a daily basis. If more than one hundred milligrams are required they are called major minerals; if we need less than one hundred milligrams, they are called trace elements. Calcium, phosphorus, magnesium, sodium, potassium, chlorine, and sulfur are all major minerals; the rest are trace elements.

Among these minerals, those which serve the function of tightening our bodies are unknown. No scientific research has been done. Probably it is a combination of trace minerals that bind our bones, muscles, and fat tightly together to form a strong organism.

All kinds of minerals were included in what the ancients called salt. In my opinion, we need natural sea salt which contains all of the sea minerals, after removing needless dirt and other substances.

After salt is removed from a concentration pond or evaporating pot, a bitter water remains that salt-makers call bittern. Magnesium is the main component, but many other sea minerals are included. This is one of the important materials in the chemical industry. On the whole, it is slightly toxic, not good to take in large amounts, but since the taste is bitter, no one wants to drink it. The sea minerals found in bittern attach to the surface of the salt crystals and enter our body with a salt content of about 0.05 percent of the salt's weight. Such a small amount may appear insignificant, but still the good effects of minerals are considerable.

Small amounts of sea minerals make salt taste better and also give the salt a better preserving effect for storing food. Even though it sounds like a contradiction, the bitter flavor enhances the taste of food, comparable to the way a small amount of salt in sweet baked goods produces a sweeter taste on the tongue.

Unfortunately, this good salt absorbs moisture from the air very easily exactly the opposite of "when it rains, it pours." Even in dry weather the salt retains moisture and will cake if kept for a long time. A small amount of sea minerals attached to the surface of the salt attracts a great deal of water, maybe up to 5 percent of the salt's weight.

Please pay attention to this point: This kind of salt has a much stronger ability to hold water, even after being ingested and inside the blood or tissues. Thus, a smaller amount of salt is needed by the body to maintain the same amount of water, making it much easier to prevent dehydration.

About Mineral Calcium

We definitely need an organic form of calcium taken from plants and sea vegetables. This form of calcium can move through the body easily; when necessary, this free-moving calcium can stay to form bones or teeth, whereas calcium derived from a mineral source can lead to the formation of stones and calcium deposits in the bones and joints.

Much of our natural water (and natural sea salt) contains small amounts of mineral calcium. The amounts are calculated in ppm (one-millionth of a gram). If the calcium content is over one hundred ppm, it is called hard water; if less than one hundred ppm, soft water. Such a small amount of calcium, as in soft water, is considered beneficial to our health. The same is true for magnesium, sulfur, and other essential minerals. In some areas natural water contains up to two thousand ppm or more of calcium; one may boil this water and the calcium will sink and stay at the bottom of the pot. Sea water also contains a lot of calcium. This is in excess of our normal needs.

Toxic Elements

New discoveries have shown that many trace elements are essential for health. It may appear strange to us that among these elements we need toxic elements such as aluminum, arsenic, fluorine, cobalt, molybdenum, and others. This research is so recent that many questions about the subject remain unanswered, such as why we need such strong poisons. Some researchers think certain elements help the body fight against invading microbes; often these are called medicinal trace elements. Not only trace elements but also some of the major minerals are toxic in large amounts. Then the question is, how do we get just the right amounts of these minerals and avoid excess? Probably the right balance here is to be found only in natural sea salt, another reason why the quality of salt is crucially important. In the urgency of new epidemics we have no time to wait until scientific research is completed.

To Obtain the Best Salt

When sea water is sun-dried over clay beds (as is still done in parts of Europe), or cooked by low fire to a concentrate, dirt will float to the surface of the water. This is mainly protein, probably from dead sea organisms, and should be removed. Then, the water becomes about 10 percent salt brine. The white clay-like material which sinks to the bottom is lime, mainly calcium, and also is not necessary; it is removed too. The salt concentration then reaches more than 26 percent and the salt begins to crystallize on the surface of the water; this is good salt. But since it is made outdoors on a salt bed, some sand and dust come in, so once more these are removed. Still, trace amounts of minerals remain attached to the salt crystals, and this is the best salt.

Today in this country, some health food stores carry different kinds of natural sea salt, most of it imported from foreign countries such as Mexico, England, France, Spain, Israel, the Phillipines, and others. The price ranges from three to ten dollars per pound – many times the grocery store price. But, compared to the price of gold, this is almost nothing. For those who buy high quality salt, their health seems more important than any amount of money, and this is right. Unfortunately, the quality varies. Some looks good and others does not. Grey salt is too dirty and some salts are completely dry. As long as good quality salt is unavailable for millions of people, I cannot recommend salt in the prevention of AIDS and other diseases. I hope the government will change the law as soon as possible. All I can say for now is, for a while, use regular commercial salt if you must. This is inevitable.

Salt and Nutrition

Through many trials and errors, nutritional research has

developed so much during the last hundred years. From an emphasis on three nutrients to the study of vitamins, minerals, and enzymes, many things have become clear. At this point we can try to look from the view of modern nutritional theories. In Table 10, I have chosen one example from five of the most common American foods – one pound each per day of meat, bread, salad, side dish, and dessert. Of course, everybody eats many different foods in combination, but for simplicity and easy calculation I have taken some typical samples from each food group. In calculating a wider variety of foods, the results may not be so different.

As you can see, the typical American diet does not contain sufficient minerals. The essential minerals, sodium, calcium, magnesium, sulfur and chlorine, are especially deficient. To cover this shortage you would have to eat a hundred pounds of carrots, which is impossible. Even if you were to mix two eggs and chicken or fish (totaling one pound) as a substitute for the beef, and ten kinds of vegetables for the lettuce, these combinations would never create balance. If you add cake and ice cream, the result is even worse. The chlorine deficiency is particularly extreme.

Now try the combinations listed in Table 11. Instead of one pound of beef, substitute a pound of brown rice; take away the apple and add a third of a pound of sunflower seeds and ten grams of salt. Ten grams of salt contains almost four thousand mg of sodium and six thousand mg of chlorine by weight. These recommendations make perfect balance. Instead of brown rice, you can use other grains such as wheat or barley; in place of sunflower seeds, other seeds, nuts, or beans will also provide good balance. Adding two ounces of sea vegetables makes even better balance.

One American doctor wrote: "If malnutrition means unbalanced nutrition, the worst malnutrition in the world is found in America." I agree. This state of malnutrition is the basis of the immuno-suppression factor in AIDS and is one of the most important co-factors in the development of the disease. For Americans who have been eating nutritionally unbalanced foods over a long

Table 10. Nutritional Content of Common Foods[8]

	Bread	Beef	Potato	Apple	Lettuce	Total	RDA	Excess /Short
Water	36.4	48.3	75.1	84.4	95.1	-	-	-
Protein	40.9	66.6	9.0	0.9	6.4	122.8	56.0	+66.8
Carbohydrate	11.7	-0-	0.4	2.7	0.9	15.7	87.0	-71.3
Fat	221.8	162.9	94.9	65.2	11.2	556.0	390.0	+166.0
Potassium (K)	1152.0	1665.0	2263.5	495.0	1188.0	6765.0	5625.0	+1140.0
Sodium (Na)	2412.0	270.8	18.0	4.5	36.0	2741.3	3300.0	-559.7
Calcium (Ca)	378.0	36.0	40.5	31.5	115.7	601.7	800.0	-199.3
Magnesium (Mg)	6.3	6.3	22.0	36.4	18.9	89.9	350.0	-260.1
Iron (Fe)	10.3	9.9	3.1	1.3	9.0	33.6	10.0	+23.6
Phosphorous (Ph)	1143.0	612.0	292.5	45.0	117.0	2209.5	800.0	+1409.5
Sulfur (Su)	NA	14.4	29.2	27.4	31.0	102.0	none	-
Chlorine (Cl)	NA	12.1	13.9	-0-	17.1	43.1	5100.0	-5056.9

Water, protein, carbohydrate, and fat = grams per pound; minerals = milligrams per pound.
Bread: commercial whole wheat with 2% nonfat dry milk and some salt. Beef: loin, choice grade.
Potato: baked. Apple: raw. Lettuce: Butterhead varieties.

The RDA for sulfur has not been established since it is always found with protein.

Table 11. Nutritional Content of Foods Based on
the Author's Recommendations[9]

	Bread	Rice	Potato	Sun-flower Seeds	Lettuce	Total	RDA	Excess/Short
Water	36.4	12.0	75.1	4.8	95.1	–	–	–
Protein	40.9	33.7	9.0	36.0	6.4	125.0	56.0	+69.0
Carbohydrate	11.7	8.5	0.4	70.9	0.9	92.4	87.0	+5.4
Fat	221.8	8.0	94.9	29.8	11.2	365.7	390.0	-24.3
Potassium (K)	1152.0	976.0	2263.5	1387.0	1188.0	6499.5	5625.0	+874.5
Sodium (Na)	2412.0	40.5	18.0	45.0	36.0	6587.5	3300.0	+3287.5
Calcium (Ca)	378.0	144.0	40.5	180.0	115.7	858.2	800.0	+58.2
Magnesium (Mg)	6.3	261.0	22.0	57.0	18.9	365.2	350.0	+15.2
Iron (Fe)	10.3	7.2	3.1	10.6	9.0	40.2	10.0	+30.2
Phosphorous (Ph)	1143.0	994.5	292.5	1255.0	117.0	3802.0	800.0	+3002.0
Sulfur (Su)	NA	NA	29.2	NA	31.0	60.2	none	–
Chlorine (Cl)	NA	NA	13.9	NA	17.1	6000.0	5100.0	+900.0

Water, protein, carbohydrate, and fat = grams per pound; minerals = milligrams per pound.
Bread, potato, and lettuce: as in Table 10. Brown rice: commercial variety.
Sunflower seeds: one-third pound only.

Ten grams of salt have been added in the calculations.

period, a perfectly balanced diet is necessary for a while in order to recover quickly. We saw that Asian descendants have the lowest incidence of AIDS. What is the main difference? In most cases, they are eating their traditional foods – mainly grains, vegetables, small amounts of fish and animal foods, and a fairly high salt content. Actually, their diet is not perfect; for example, they eat white rice, white bread, and some cakes and candies. But still they show better health results.

Salt Deficiency and AIDS

Since I learned more than fifty years ago that typical tuberculosis (weight loss, night sweating, afternoon slight fevers, cough, etc.) is related to salt deficiency, I have been observing sick people very carefully. Now I am certain there is also a relationship between AIDS and salt deficiency. After studying the minerals, I understand why. Such crucially important minerals as calcium, potassium, sodium, chlorine, magnesium, and a minimum amount of trace elements are missing from the American diet. Chlorine especially is an important element for killing the causative microbes of disease and for cleansing the body. There is no other way to get enough chlorine except through natural salt. Still the problem is not resolved, for as long as you are eating meat, it is difficult to obtain enough natural salt for healing because while your sodium requirements are being met, there is not enough chlorine. Before you begin to use more salt in your cooking, at least one week of a strict vegetarian diet is recommended. It is good to eat raw vegetables, but with caution, for if you have had large amounts of sugar or fruit but not much animal food, raw vegetables are not necessary. Please read the later chapters carefully for more on plant and animal foods.

Chapter 9

Chewing

Healing power, a strong immune system, and body rejuvenation are all enhanced by good chewing. This subject should be at the beginning of a book about the prevention of AIDS, but I know that modern-day people are busy and if I had put this first, many would have decided with just one glance not to read this book. Chewing is not a subject that satisfies intellectual curiosity; it is a matter of practice.

I have written so many things about good food selection, but if you don't chew your food very well, even good food does not work as you would expect. Not only grandmothers from ancient times, but also many wise men have taught and have made recommendations about chewing. In the Essene Gospel of John found in the Dead Sea Scrolls, Jesus suggests: "And chew well your food with your teeth, that it become water, and that the angel of water turn it into blood in your body. And eat slowly, as if it were a prayer you make to the Lord." Leonardo da Vinci, super-genius of the Renaissance, recommended this practice and, closer to modern times, Prime Minister William Gladstone of Great Britain asserted that "you cannot be a great man unless you chew each mouthful of food at least thirty-two times." (The number thirty-two correlates with our thirty-two teeth.)

Mahatma Gandhi advised, "Chew your drink and drink your food"; his was a reminder that we must not simply swallow our food. Chew your food until it becomes like a liquid and drink this as you would water. Even water you have to chew; don't gulp it.

Even prior to Gandhi's influence, America had a great predecessor in this field, William Horace Fletcher (1849-1919), although his name is not even mentioned in the *Encyclopedia Britannica*. Fletcher began endorsing this practice ("Fletcherism") around the end of the nineteenth century. Within ten years he had become famous, not only in this country, but also in Europe and Japan and probably throughout the world millions of people followed his teaching. Fletcher was the first person to approach the importance of chewing for health and longevity with a scientific attitude. "Chewing increases immunity and cures alcoholism" was one of his statements, and this is so important now for those suffering from AIDS.

As often happens with revolutionary thinkers, Fletcher was attacked for his mistakes and his name disappeared; I feel the time has come for a revival of his ideas, with some corrections in his nutritional theory, for he did not necessarily recommend whole grains or whole wheat bread. He also allowed people to spit out the unliquidified stuff after mastication, and this was his biggest mistake because it causes constipation. Still, there are many things we can learn from him.

Fletcher himself experienced the effects of chewing well. While in his 40s, his body was aging, he was overweight, his hair had turned white, and he was always tired. He started his new research. He understood that health depends on nutrition, that nutrition comes from the food we eat, and that the mouth is the entrance of food. Further, chewing is the first step in digestion. Thus, he started his study from the mouth through the process of chewing and the action of saliva. At the same time he began chewing very well and found that many troubles were resolved just by this practice. He began teaching. He was also a famous athlete and successful in business.

Dr. Russell Chittenden, a professor at Yale University, worked with Fletcher and contributed much to medical and nutritional knowledge. For example, at that time the commonly accepted protein requirement for one person per day was 120 grams. Dr. Chittenden claimed that our requirement should be 40 grams a day. Recently the World Health Organization tentatively determined the requirement to be 37 grams a day.

After five months of trial, Fletcher wrote, "My head was clear, my body felt springy. I enjoyed walking. I had not had a single cold for five months." He also lost about fifty pounds and his athletic abilities returned. He looked like a young man and many people expected him to live over a hundred years. However, he died suddenly at the age of sixty-nine; it was not a short life, but probably his opponents attacked him, claiming it was his fault that he died. His name, organization, and teachings suddenly disappeared. His mistakes were that he did not recommend whole grains and that he allowed people to spit out the roughage. Also, his hard athletic training shortened his life, the reasons for which will be discussed in the lifestyle chapter.

Fast Food, Quick Eating

Quick eating is a modern-day fad. Everyone is so busy and has no time to cook. Even at restaurants one must wait some thirty minutes to be served, so people think it's better to go to a fast food place where the food is ready in a few minutes. The food is prepared for gulping.

The taste is good, the nutrition is okay, and protein, fat, and carbohydrates are all in there. At least this is what the advertisers tell us. The food melts in your mouth with any beverage and becomes creamy and easy to swallow. The food also has a nice aroma and is beautiful looking. The modern food industry has developed so much.

Just look at America's favorite foods: white bread, muffins, doughnuts, croissants, waffles, chiffon, popovers, cream puffs, angelfood cake, etc. Also, juices and many beverages ready to gulp. Another favorite food is hamburger, ground and prepared so that people can bolt it down. It seems that much chewing time is being saved. But this is not a good way to eat.

Chewing and Digestion

As Horace Fletcher stated, a magical healing power comes from chewing. Let us now review the functions of chewing.

1. Chewing breaks down food. Solid foods must be broken down into tiny pieces as much as possible. No one can swallow a Brazil nut whole. Even peanuts or pumpkin seeds, if swallowed whole, will create problems in the throat and the stomach. An unchewed chunk of meat stuck in the throat has even been the cause of death. Meat cannot be easily swallowed or mixed by digestive juices in the stomach if it is not well-chewed. Foods must be broken down and mixed with saliva.

A large portion of our diet is composed of carbohydrates, but there are two kinds of carbohydrates, each of which is treated differently by our bodies. Grains, seeds, and nuts are our most important foods; they are brought to the central area of the mouth where they must be well chewed. It is in this area that abundant amounts of saliva are secreted. This saliva contains the digestive enzyme ptyalin which breaks down the complex carbohydrates into simple sugar, which in turn converts to glucose. If the carbohydrate we take in is a simple sugar, it is processed at the tip of the tongue, diluted with saliva, and swallowed without chewing.

If we do not chew well, the ptyalin enzyme cannot permeate the grains and the starch does not change into glucose. The stomach has no digestive juices for the breakdown of carbohydrates; it is more like a fermentation tank, but if there is no ptyalin mixed with the carbohydrates, this fermentation cannot take place. The result will be a feeling of discomfort in the stomach along with excessive gas. The pancreas does produce some digestive enzymes, but not in sufficient amounts – the undigested food goes down to the very end of the digestive tract. You can test this by swallowing a couple of grains of cooked corn and checking your stool the next day. You will find them whole and undigested.

2. Chewing activates the whole digestive system. Chewing our food has a positive effect on the other digestive processes, so that the activity performed in the mouth and by the jaws stimulates the stomach, intestines, and all the digestive organs. The pancreas produces more digestive juice, the liver sends more bile to the duodenum, and so on.

Also, chewing relaxes the body. We need to eat without hurrying. A relaxed condition helps digestion, and chewing helps to produce this condition both physically and psychologically.

3. Chewing increases the production of saliva. We see that saliva is important for digestion, but its good effects go far beyond that. We have three pairs of salivary glands, a total of six. Different foods and tastes draw out different salivas from different glands. The parotid glands are located under the ears on both sides; they are much larger than the other glands and produce the greatest amount of saliva. When we use our molars, the parotid glands produce a saliva rich in ptyalin to digest carbohydrates. Salty and bitter foods also stimulate these glands. The submaxillary glands are located along the side of the lower jaw bone. They produce additional saliva needed for sour and oily foods, and for chewing meat. The sublingual glands are smaller, situated at the floor of the mouth. When we eat sweet foods or bite into fruits and vegetables these glands produce a thinner saliva to dilute strong sweet tastes.

Even when we're not eating, a small amount of saliva is constantly produced to keep moisture in the mouth. These supplies of saliva are like fountains which are never dry, but which at times may stop their flow. If our body loses water or if the percentage of water content decreases, the production of saliva, too, will drop; if this continues to the point of stopping temporarily, the mouth will dry up and we feel thirsty.

4. Chewing improves the taste of food. Further, each bite of

food has three tastes – beginning taste, middle taste, and end taste. Through the careful practice of chewing you will be able to distinguish and enjoy all three tastes. The true taste of food is in the end taste, the best taste of all. Whole grains have the best taste for everyone without exception, but most people are not aware of this because they have never chewed grains so thoroughly. Try it today. Many kinds of gourmet food taste good for the first second, but have no taste at all if chewed. Enjoy your food by chewing slowly for a long time.

5. Chewing makes for good food selection. "One man's meat is another man's poison." "There's no arguing about taste." These common sayings indicate that liking or disliking certain foods is purely an individual matter. I do not believe any such thing. Our choice of food is mainly based on habit and acquired knowledge. Each culture has some kind of food tradition. We grow up with such foods and this habit is difficult to break. We want stability when it comes to food.

But at the same time, somehow we grow tired of the same food every day and we want variety. This kind of contradiction always exists in humans and the natural world. If occasionally we eat exotic food, we often think the taste is wonderful. Often, new ideas come from nutritional research, education, or advertisements and these become our favorite foods. But if we chew our food well, our taste returns to the natural state. You will find that each individual is not that different, that a minimum amount of meat satisfies your appetite, and that you lose interest in highly processed foods. Furthermore, in today's world, sometimes food contains poison or toxic materials by accident or mistake and swallowing the food is dangerous. If you chew well, the strange taste gives a warning and the bad food can be spat out before swallowing. Already we have seen many cases of this happening.

6. Chewing prevents overeating. Diabetes, obesity, and many other diseases are related to overeating; one of the most difficult problems is how we can control this excessive appetite. The stomach

is a flexible organ; its capacity cannot determine optimum food volume, as it can hold even twice as much food as normal capacity in an emergency. Food is essential for sustaining our life and activity, but how much is enough and how much is too much? Beyond our knowledge or thinking, our body knows. We don't need large amounts of food to maintain good health and activities. To control a big appetite and to prevent disease, chewing is definitely important. If we chew well, the stomach feels full when it is at 80-90 percent of its capacity. This is the best way to maintain good health. Mental workers who engage in little physical activity can feel full when the stomach is 70-80 percent full. If we can start working or thinking soon after each meal without taking rest or a nap, we are probably eating a proper amount. This practice also saves a lot of food.

For weight loss, I recommend chewing twice as much. The safest way to expel excess water from the overweight body is through saliva – again, by chewing well. To do this, it is good to endure a slight thirst; instead of drinking water, the extra saliva combines with food and goes back to the body. If you don't lose weight you are not chewing enough; chew three times as much. If you still have no improvement, chew your food four times as much. Surely you can lose weight.

7. Chewing safeguards against diseases. The most common cause of stomach disease is rather simple: overeating; swallowing big pieces of food; using strong spices; too much sugar, alcohol, coffee, or salt; very hot soup or tea; alcohol; midnight eating – all of these are related to improper eating habits, especially in the matter of chewing. If we eat without chewing well, big pieces of food remain in the stomach for a long time and the stomach excretes more acid and makes for improper fermentation resulting in bad gas, belches, and burps. From such small problems real stomach troubles begin. Breads and other kinds of spongy foods need a lot of chewing to expel all the air; if not, more gas will be the result.

The main part of the small intestine is well designed for choosing and absorbing only good and well-digested food and for pushing along the undigested matter, so that diseases of the small intestine are relatively rare.

All kinds of unfavorable foods are sent to the colon, so that colon troubles, of which there are many kinds, are the most complex problems. For handling such unwanted substances, dietary fiber is favorable for the colon, but undigested chunks of meat are not good, because protein-decomposing microbes, which can damage the intestinal wall and other body tissues, also may increase.

Cholera, dysentery, and typhoid bacteria come in via the mouth and cause digestive diseases. The polio and hepatitis viruses also invade from the mouth. Even the strong hydrochloric acid in the stomach cannot penetrate into big pieces of food. They must be chewed, as saliva has a special property which kills invading microbes from food.[1]

8. Chewing adjusts the water content of foods. About 70 percent of our body is water. Foods vary considerably in the percentage of their water content, but by the time they reach the end of the digestive tract their water content is almost the same as the body's. Our mouth is made for the purpose of adjusting this fluid content. If this is not equalized in the mouth, the food can be harmful to the stomach and the intestine. Cooked grains, for example, contain about 70 percent water. Since this matches the bodily percentage, there is little problem in digesting grains. Meat has about 45 percent water, so we have to add another 25 percent in saliva. To be more exact, meat has a high content of protein and fat and these should be diluted much more than carbohydrates. Only chewing can adjust this needed dilution. Roasted peanuts have only 5 percent water or less, so another 65 percent must be added. Peanuts have to be chewed very well, otherwise the stomach will suffer.

Vegetables and fruits, on the other hand, contain 85 to 95 percent water, so if we don't chew them they will quickly fill the stomach and leave no room for other foods. But if we chew them well, the juice is extracted in the mouth, thus passing easily through the stomach within ten to fifteen minutes.

Coffee is about 97 to 99 percent water, but if we drink it at the 97 percent consistency, it is much too strong for the body and needs to be further diluted. If not, it will tend to irritate the surface of the stomach and possibly lead to stomach trouble. Although plain water or milk can dilute strong coffee, the best thing is still saliva. The same may be said for vinegar and alcoholic drinks. Sugar, salt, and many spices contain a little water, but more is needed to dilute them; otherwise, they irritate the mucous membranes which line the mouth, throat, and stomach. So, in effect, almost everything is potentially harmful. What percentage is good, no one knows; only the tongue can determine, and saliva can help.

9. As we gain strength through training and exercise, chewing strengthens the teeth and gums. Since teeth are the most important tools for chewing, good teeth are the basis of health and longevity. Develop strong teeth and keep them throughout your life. Your aim should be to not lose even one tooth. Retaining one's teeth is also a sign of a young body. The teeth and gums are kept strong not only through training and exercise, but through the saliva which excretes a special hormone for maintaining strong teeth. The gums support the teeth, so strong gums are the prerequisite for developing strong teeth.

10. Chewing makes the body younger. The special hormone, parotin, is produced only by the parotid glands. This hormone is absorbed by the lymph vessels through the mouth during chewing and then it goes into the bloodstream. If it goes down to the stomach with food, it is destroyed by gastric juices. This is a unique hormone. Parotin stimulates cell metabolism and thus renews the entire body. Our metabolism slows down with age, at a rate that differs from person to person, but if we can keep this renewing process always going, we do not age as markedly and can live many years longer. Good examples of this are the Hunza and Andes mountain people who live to very advanced ages. They chew their food very well.[2]

This rejuvenation effect has been demonstrated through the medical research done by Dr. Tomozaburo Ogata, professor at the School of Medicine, Tokyo University. With his colleagues, Dr. Ogata proved this special quality of the hormone parotin and its effect on rejuvenation. They were able to clarify the entire mechanism of how it is secreted and absorbed. Ogata also processed parotin from cow's saliva into a drug which he injected into a number of elderly people. By this treatment all the subjects ended up looking ten years younger. However, by repeated use this drug would become less effective and finally would not work at all, just as insulin injections eventually fail to halt the progress of diabetes. Also, a few people had some allergic reactions. There is no golden road for health and longevity; we have to produce this for ourselves.

11. Chewing increases T-cells. Finally, we come to the most important point of all. One of the special effects of parotin is to stimulate the thymus gland, thereby producing more T-cells. These are one type of white blood cell (lymphocyte) which is essential in the fight against causative agents of infection. It is said that the AIDS virus attacks the T-cells, making them their hosts and stealing from them the nutrition needed for reproducing the virus. As a result the increased numbers of the virus spread widely and invade many other T-cells. If the T-cells are overcome by the AIDS virus, they lose their power.

The thymus gland is a unique organ of the body. Other organs and glands develop in the body along with the body's growth, but with the thymus it is just the opposite: it is at its most developed stage in the newborn baby and in the first year of life. As the body grows, the thymus does not grow; in puberty it shrinks. The function of the thymus gland was unknown until the last few decades. Just recently some of its functions have become clear and many interesting observations have been reported. One of its most important functions has to do with the immune system. The thymus gland seems to have the ability to give a special training to stem cells (immature white blood cells), making them into T-cells, or T-lymphocytes. Still now so many things are unknown about the thymus, but its function in the immune system is an established theory in the medical world. Not many people have yet paid much attention to the relationship between the thymus gland and the hormone parotin. The *American Medical Dictionary* states, "In rabbits it [parotin] affects the leukocyte count."[3] It seems that this is not yet proven in human testing, but if you try to increase parotin through better chewing, you can actually find that you are stronger against infections.

Eat Slowly

Perhaps now you can understand the importance of chewing and why you have to do it. Here are some estimates for the time needed for chewing at each meal:

- For healthy people, about fifty times, which means about thirty minutes per meal; if talking time is included, you need an hour or more as you wish.
- If you have some health problems, you should chew each bite a hundred times or more; this will take about an hour just for chewing.
- If you are seriously ill, try to chew two hundred times or more and take at least two hours for your meal. This amount of chewing is needed in order for parotin to be produced from the saliva and absorbed into your bloodstream.

Even chewing gum is good for this purpose, provided it contains no sugar or chemicals. At one time chewing gum was very popular, but now it has almost been forgotten.

Now I have to say something that may seem a little strange. The recommendations above are for daily practice. But occasionally – once a week or once a month, whatever you wish to try – it may be good to chew less, as you may be doing now. Otherwise, the stomach and intestines could become lazy, over-protected, and too sensitive should an emergency situation occur. If this contradiction sounds strange, let us examine whether anything is 100 percent pure in this world or in our daily lives, unless it is made by humans, such as refined sugar and salt. It seems natural that there are always some exceptions and mixtures.

But if you make better chewing a part of your daily practice, there will be clear improvements in your health and in your natural immunity.

Chapter 10

The Microbe Kingdom

AIDS and the opportunistic diseases that characterize it are caused by viruses and various bacteria, fungi, protozoa, and others, so it would be good to understand a little more about microbes.

The Invisible World

Even in ancient times, some thinkers had the notion that tiny living things existed in the air, water, soil, and in the body. For example, Aristotle described the sperm and the ovum, which were invisible to the naked eye; Marcus Varro (116-27 B.C.?) mentioned microorganisms; and Lucretius (99-55 B.C.?) expressed the view that "the plague must be caused by a kind of atom." In the sixteenth century one marvelous man appeared, Girolamo Fracastoro (1478-1553). A friend of Copernicus and an astronomer in his own right, Fracastoro was also a renowned physician and the author of a famous poem entitled "Syphilis, or the French Disease." In his book, *On Contagion and Contagious Diseases*, (1546) Fracastoro stated that minute, rapidly multiplying bodies are transferred from an infected person to another person. He came to this conclusion simply by means of observation and imagination. This was the first step of scientific bacteriology, but unfortunately his opinion and his name soon fell into disrepute due to the fame of another physician, Paracelsus.

The Chinese character for the wind and the common cold is the same (風). This is a combination of two characters, one of which represents 'everything' (凡) and the other, 'worm' (虫). This indicates that the wind and/or the common cold were understood by ancient peoples to be filled with some life form that no one could see, a concept probably dating from about 1,000 B.C.

The Invisible Becomes Visible

In 1590 the Dutch spectacle-maker Zacharias Janssen (1580-1638) and his father made the first microscope by combining two lenses. In 1608 he constructed a telescope with the help of his fellow eyeglass-maker, Hans Lippershey, who popularized the invention throughout Europe. Galileo heard about the design and made his own telescope and microscope, receiving much more public interest and support for the telescope. In 1661 Marcello Malpighi (1628-94) reported the discovery of blood capillaries seen through the microscope, but he had not yet been able to see bacteria. Malpighi was a professor at the University of Bologna and became the Pope's chief physician. He is considered to be the founder of microscopic anatomy.

Another Dutchman, Anton van Leeuwenhoek (1632-1723) made the best microscope in the world at that time. Not a physician or scientist, he was a cloth merchant with little scientific education who so excelled in his hobby of grinding lenses that he was able to fashion an instrument with a magnification power of 270. By means of his homemade lenses van Leeuwenhoek became the first person to catch a glimpse into a new world that had been only imagined for hundreds of years prior to his time. In countless microscopic studies he made observations and notes on various forms of bacteria (which he called animalcula, or little animals) - spiral (spirilla), rod-shaped (bacilla), and spherical (coccal) - and pictured their arrangement in infected material. With his instrument van Leeuwenhoek was also able to demonstrate the entire life cycle of small insects and how they breed in and around other living things. He gave the first definitive account of the red blood cell, discovered sperm cells, and demonstrated the existence of the capillary connections between arteries and veins. For these studies van Leeuwenhoek is known as the father of both bacteriology and scientific microscopy. He became quite famous and was visited by such notables as the Queen of England and Peter the Great of Russia.

Van Leeuwenhoek's work is perhaps more significant than Columbus's discovery of the New World or the Copernican theory of heliocentricity, because the world of microorganisms is as wideranging and deeply integral to our survival as the existence of air and water. We cannot even think about modern biology, physiology, genetics, agriculture, or industrial research without taking microscopy into consideration. But it seems strange that for two hundred years after his discoveries the scientific and medical establishment has paid little attention to van Leeuwenhoek's work.

Scientists, Microbes, and Disease

The great French scholar Louis Pasteur (1822-1895), considered the father of our modern scientific medicine, was also not a physician by training. A chemist by profession, Pasteur became known for his experiments with the fermentation of wine and other foods, research which demonstrated that microbes were responsible for the fermentation process. In his studies he also discovered that these same microbes were responsible for the spoilage and putrefaction of foods, and he proceeded to develop his process of pasteurization to preserve foods, a process still in use to this day. Pasteur also ushered in the age of modern bacteriology by isolating the bacteria related to silkworm diseases and demonstrating a method for preventing contagion. He succeeded in developing vaccinations for sheep anthrax and chicken cholera and in 1885 also saved the lives of some people who had been bitten by a rabid dog.

Robert Koch (1843-1910) was twenty-one years younger than Pasteur, but he started early in his career to research microbes and their relationship to disease. In 1882 he discovered *Mycobacterium tuberculosis,* the bacteria associated with tuberculosis, which at that time was one of the most deadly and feared of all diseases. He later showed this bacteria through a microscope to the famous Hungarian dermatologist, Moriz Kaposi, whose name the AIDS crisis has brought to the forefront by way of the syndrome known as Kaposi's sarcoma. At the time Kaposi strongly denied that what he was shown could cause disease. In 1883 Koch discovered, isolated, and cultured another bacteria, *Vibrio cholerae,* the one responsible for cholera. He showed this to a colleague named Pettenkopfel, who, like Kaposi, argued that the bacteria could not possibly be the cause of the disease. To prove his point, Pettenkopfel drank an entire glass of the cholera bacteria that Koch had cultivated and did not get the disease. Despite this astounding demonstration, most people supported Koch's ideas, and he went on to establish the foundations of modern microbiology.

Most Microbes Are Helpful

To date about fifty thousand species of bacteria have been classified, but less than one hundred of these have been linked to disease. The most plentiful species in the world are the fungi, including yeasts and molds. About one hundred thousand kinds have been identified, but of these, again, only about one hundred affect humans. Of these one hundred, about twenty can be the cause of fatal diseases, while forty-five can cause superficial infections of the skin or mucous membranes.

Thus we can say that, except for a few, most bacteria are not only harmless, but are constantly at work keeping us and our entire planet alive and well. Without them we could not exist. For example, our drinking water should be free of bacteria, but in fact it is both impossible and unnecessary to remove or kill them completely. If a milliliter of water contains five hundred microorganisms or fewer, it is considered to be good water for drinking. A square inch of grassland soil contains as many as a million microbes, in some places more, in others less, depending on the available nutrition and water content. The human body always carries billions of microbes, mainly in the large intestine but also in the mouth, throat, nose, the surface of the skin, and many other places. Many of these tiny organisms help us to stay healthy.

Nutrition and Environment for Microbes

Generally, microbes need protein, fat, and carbohydrates for growth, and some kinds of microbes need minerals such as calcium, sulfur, phosphorous, potassium, iron, etc. – almost the same requirements as for our body cells. If microbes are to multiply, a certain temperature needs to be maintained, usually about 98° F, almost the same as for our body; some can resist colder temperatures, and a few can survive greater heat. Most microbes cannot tolerate light, especially the violet and ultraviolet rays, although some species can live under strong sunshine. Microbes are dormant in dry environments and cannot multiply, but if they find food, it will contain sufficient water so that they can absorb both water and nutrients.

Microbes generally do not tolerate chemicals or acidic or alkaline conditions, but there are exceptions, too; some do well under acidic conditions, others prefer an alkaline environment. The majority of microbes live at a pH of 6 to 7, slightly more on the acid side than our blood. (See the chapter on acid/alkaline balance.) Fungi tolerate acid well and prefer sugars for their nutritional needs.

But certain microorganisms seem to possess a magic power that enables them to resist an environment that is harmful to them. They do this by converting into spore forms and lying dormant until the environment changes again to one that they can tolerate. For many years they can live in this spore form, and then change back to active bacteria.

Many microbes require oxygen for life, but some prefer carbon dioxide. Like plants, they return oxygen to the air. Others have the ability to convert nitrogen gas into soluble form in a water environment, a characteristic known as nitrogen fixation. Still others can decompose proteins and nitrates and convert them into gases.

Powerful Kingdom

If we consider all these kinds of microbes living and working together as a whole, they almost seem almighty, as if nothing is impossible to them. Their power comes from a remarkable ability to reproduce. Some can duplicate and double their numbers within a time span of twenty minutes. With sufficient nutrients, some can grow from one to a trillion within ten hours. If we ask why they increase so much, we must also wonder why five billion humans now cover the earth; it seems all living organisms of this world want to increase. Generally, the smaller ones increase faster than larger ones.

Most animals cannot digest cellulose, the main part of trees and the woody part of vegetables, but microbes can take nutrients from cellulose and decompose the material into simpler forms. This same ability enables them to decompose animal excretions and the dead bodies of animals and plants, and return this matter to the soil. Without this service our world would be submerged under dead bodies and fallen leaves within a few years. Microbes are great scavengers. They can even neutralize poisons as well as organic materials; they die in the poison but others increase again. After all the atomic bomb explosions, hydrogen bomb tests, and nuclear accidents of our time, the world is less polluted by radiation than was feared. New research is indicating that microbes are even cleaning up the radiation.

The Smallest Microbes

After World War II the Germans developed the electron microscope which has the capacity of magnifying up to 200,000 times or more. The most powerful compound light microscopes can magnify only 2,000 times. Now, microscopes can magnify more than one million times. Once this powerful new tool was put to use, one of the many things that became clear was that viruses were found to be living microbes since they contain genes and can multiply.

The concept of viruses dates from the last century, and the diseases caused by them have been known since older times. Whether viruses are living organisms or not was not known. But understanding how such minute microorganisms are causative agents of disease is quite new. Viruses are so small that they can pass through porcelain filters; thus they are called filterable agents. Unlike bacteria, viruses cannot live independently of their host cells, whether animal or plant cells, or other bacteria. Viruses take their nutrition from the host cells and can multiply rapidly. A single cell parasitized by a polio virus was reported to have produced one hundred thousand polio virus particles within a few hours – a hundred times faster than bacteria can multiply. Usually viruses do not kill the host cells, for the death of the host cell means that they also would die, but not always. Viruses are attracted to attack certain host cells; neurotropic viruses affect the brain and nervous system, dermatropic viruses attack the skin, pneumotropic viruses involve the respiratory system, viscerotropic viruses harm the inside organs, etc.

We are still at the beginning stages in our understanding of viruses. In the last few decades many viruses have been discovered; hundreds are related to human diseases. How many more there are is not known. Due to the varieties of structures and life cycles, the possibilities for diseases caused by viruses are higher than in the case of bacteria or fungi.

Bacteria and all animals and plants have DNA (deoxyribonucleic acid) in their cells. The DNA carries genetic information from parent to offspring and it synthesizes RNA (ribonucleic acid), which transmits the DNA's messages to continue cell duplication and growth. But viruses, the smallest and most primitive of life forms, have either DNA or RNA, never both, in their structure. Pox, herpes, and adenoviruses are DNA viruses, and polio, flu, and rabies viruses carry only RNA.

Viruses can also invade bacteria as their host cells; this type of virus is called a bacteriophage (bacteria eater). Even smaller viruses have been discovered; they are of the RNA type and are called viroids, known to cause plant diseases, but, fortunately, no human infection has yet been reported. Recent research on viruses has uncovered ever smaller and smaller varieties, so that the field of virology has become increasingly specialized and complicated. Viruses also can mutate and easily make new strains.

One of the outcomes of bacteriological research over the past hundred years has been the discovery of antibiotics, which promised to eradicate all infectious disease, but antibiotics have no effect on viral diseases. Viruses live inside of the body cells, so it is difficult to kill the virus without destroying our body cells. One hope is effective vaccines against viral strains, but a new vaccine would be needed for each new strain, which would be difficult. No one can see what kind of virus is coming next.

Retrovirus, Lentivirus

Some of the viruses have a special enzyme, reverse transcriptase, which changes the viral RNA into DNA. These newly discovered retroviruses invade a host cell, cut the host's DNA, and connect their own viral genes. This process abnormalizes the host cells and can cause them to multiply out of control, causing leukemia or cancerous tumors. HTLV-I is this kind of virus. Among these viruses are some which infect their human or animal hosts very slowly. For example, the incubation period of many other viruses is from seven to fourteen days in some cases and from one to twelve months in others, but with the new lentiviruses (slow viruses) the incubation period can last from six months to ten years, and in some cases possibly thirty years.

HIV, the AIDS virus, is considered to belong to this class of retro- and lentiviruses. The HIV virus does not cause cancer or leukemia, but mainly invades the T-cells and can also attack brain and nerve cells directly, multiply quickly, destroy host cells, and cause mental and nervous system malfunctions. The main problem with lentiviruses is brain damage. HIV is a neurotropic virus but is also recognized as a lymphotropic virus which selectively attacks the white blood cells and the T-cells.

Vital Cycles

Our nutritional needs are provided by plants and animals as well as a small amount of minerals along with water and salt. Plants, the basis of the food chain, live by the light energy of the sun, the gaseous carbon dioxide in the air, and by absorbing water, minerals, and other nutrients from the soil. Because our body is unable to absorb mineral elements directly from the earth, we get most of our minerals from plants and also from the animals that eat these plants to meet their mineral needs. Because plants are always taking up minerals, the soil would soon become depleted if it were not somehow replenished. The earth has a plentiful supply of minerals stored up in its mountains, rocks, and stones, and a great deal of minerals are restored from the decomposition of organic matter. To a certain extent, plants can break up rocks in the soil to get their minerals, but this ability is very limited. Water and microbes help greatly in this action. When water freezes, it expands and breaks up stones and rocks into smaller and smaller pieces. Certain microbes have the ability to consume rocks and break them down into the simple minerals that plants can absorb. These microbes are essential for creating a healthy, fertile topsoil where plants can grow and become a source of minerals for animals and humans.

In a way, we can say that all kinds of animals – including humans – are the parasites of plants and that plants are the parasites of the earth, which in turn depends upon microbes for the release of its minerals. All microbes are kinds of parasites to humans, animals, plants, and minerals.

The Carbon Cycle

Carbon is one of the most basic and important elements needed by all living things. The carbon atom and its way of forming end-less combinations of molecules is the basis of what is called organic chemistry, or the chemistry of life. Plants, upon which all other life depends, can only get their carbon from the carbon dioxide (CO_2) which exists in gaseous form in the air. Since CO_2 is always in the air but in limited quantities, it must constantly be supplied. This vital supply comes from several sources, both living and non-living. One important source is the exhaled breath of all animals. But the most significant amount of CO_2 comes from the respiration of microbes.

Animals get their carbohydrates, the basic fuel of life, from plants and excrete it in the form of CO_2 as they breathe. If there were enough animals on the earth converting their food from car-bohydrates to carbon dioxide in relation to the number of plants doing the opposite, then the carbon cycle would be in perfect balance. But such is not the case. There is a lot of carbon that cannot be respired and released back into the environment as car-bon dioxide for the plants to use. Plants, and animals to a lesser extent, die with much carbon bound up in their systems. If there was no way for this carbon to be converted back into CO_2, then all plant and animal life would soon cease. Of course, we can again thank the microbe kingdom. Fungi and bacteria break up the com-plex carbon compounds in the excreta and dead material and initiate the processes of decomposition and decay. In so doing, they release CO_2 gas back into the atmosphere, keeping the plants and the carbon cycle alive.

The Nitrogen Cycle

Nitrogen is another key element in all living things since it is the foundation of the amino acids which, in turn, are the basis of all proteins. About 80 percent of the air is nitrogen, but it is not in a form plants or animals can use. To be absorbed by plants (and thus eaten by animals), nitrogen must be converted into nitrates (nitro-gen with oxygen) in the soil. Just as with CO_2 in the air, nitrates are present in the soil only in small quantities that must be constantly replenished. This is done almost entirely by the activity of microbes that live in the soil, where they decompose organic matter and convert the nitrogen in the air into nitrates.

The process of decomposition is like a mini-food chain within a larger food chain. Organic materials such as feces and dead plants are eaten by different microbes; by means of this process simpler compounds are formed, one of which is ammonia (NH_3). The ammonia is then eaten by nitrifying bacteria which convert it into nitrites. The nitrites are then consumed by still other nitrifying bacteria which convert them into nitrates. The plants then absorb these nitrates and make them into more complex nitrogen compounds (amino acids and proteins) and the cycle begins again. When gardeners and farmers work manure into the soil they are depending on this microbial process to turn organic matter into nitrates that will keep the plants well nourished and healthy.

The conversion of nitrogen in the air into a nitrate is a process called nitrogen fixation. This is a beautiful process involving two groups of organisms as well as certain species of plants. One group of bacteria lives in the soil itself, the other penetrates the cells and lives harmoniously in the root hairs of legumes such as clover, alfalfa, vetch, or soybeans. The microbes receive nourishment from these plants without harming them, eventually forming nodules filled with rapidly growing bacteria. These nodules of live, multiplying bacteria are what bind the nitrogen of the air into the nitrates which the plant then removes and uses for its own growth. Microbes in the soil fix nitrogen from the air into fertilizer and accomplish many times more than can be done artificially by all of man's chemical factories. The only other natural way of fixing nitrogen into nitrates occurs during severe electrical storms when the charge of lightning carries large amounts of free nitrogen into the soil.

Other Mineral Cycles
Essential mineral elements such as calcium, sulfur, magnesium,

potassium, boron, and others are absorbed from the soil in solution by the roots of plants. They are returned to the soil by microbial cycles as we have seen for carbon and nitrogen. As well as supporting the life of plants and animals by recycling minerals and other important elements, microbes keep our world clean and free of debris. Fallen leaves, trees, and animal bodies return to the soil and a new life cycle by virtue of the ceaseless activity of microbes.

Contamination and Purification

Bacteria also purify sewage by living on the impurities and converting them into simple and inoffensive substances. People who get their drinking water from wells benefit from this process. Water trickling through the soil is filtered by bacteria as they consume toxic matter and by the soil and other materials in the earth itself; contaminated water may emerge from deep wells in the earth practically clean and pure. This relationship is not absolute; some bacteria contaminate the water and others purify it.

We can see that the soil is an alive and active part of the food chain, and that the quality of our food and health is directly linked to the life and quality of the soil created for plants by microbes.

Microbes and Food

Since ancient times microbes have played a key role in the chemical processes of day-to-day life, especially with foods. As microorganisms work on certain foods, enzymes are produced that break down sugars and starches into various byproducts which transform the material into foods with completely different qualities of taste, color, texture, and biochemical composition.

When cow's or goat's milk is churned, butter forms as tiny globules of fat bind together with a small amount of milk solids. The residual liquid is what we call buttermilk. This residue is usually allowed to stand, souring and curdling as bacteria convert the milk sugar (lactose) into lactic acid. The conversion of sugar to an acid is the process known as ripening, the basis of many dairy products such as various cheeses, sour cream, yogurt, kefir, and so on. Normal milk bacteria present in the air are the usual agents of ripening; the best and most widely known is the genus *lactobacillus,* but there are others as well. The ripening process contributes a unique flavor, texture, and color as well as helping to preserve the various products, since the strong acidity retards the growth of other bacteria and molds which might spoil the food. Cheese is made as the curds separate from the liquid portion of milk either by bacterial fermentation (ripening) or by the action of a milk-curdling enzyme (rennin) that is taken from the stomachs of calves.

We can imagine that the first alcoholic beverage was probably discovered when one of our thirsty ancestors drank some old juice that had been sitting around for awhile. Today, alcoholic beverages are made by the fermenting abilities of certain microbes (we call them yeasts) found in a mash of fruit or grain. Wine is made from grape juice, cider from apple juice, and beer from a blend of grains. The microbes consume the sugars (carbohydrates) from these various liquids thus producing alcohol, which is a compound of carbon, hydrogen, and oxygen.

From Daily Bread to Medicine

Bread baking is similar to the production of alcohol in that microbial yeasts are breaking down sugars to form carbon dioxide and alcohol. Here, carbon dioxide forms bubbles that cause the dough to lighten (leaven) or rise. When the dough is baked the alcohol evaporates away, the carbon dioxide expands and is driven off, and we have a risen loaf. For many centuries bread was made by the use of a small amount of live dough (starter) saved from one batch to the next, often for many years, or by allowing well-kneaded dough to sit for several hours in a warm place to obtain a similar result. (There was never any yeast added.) Adding commercial yeast to breads is a practice that has grown only in recent years, since the refining of flour made the dough lifeless and unable to support the activity of natural yeasts everpresent in the air. To make naturally leavened bread the flour must be freshly milled in a low-temperature mill (slow grinding stones) to preserve the nutrients that the naturally-occurring airborne yeasts need to do their leavening work. If you have never tasted this kind of bread, try to find some or make some of your own. This is the real staff of life that our ancestors produced for thousands of years. There is no comparison in terms of taste and good nutrition.

Microbes also produce a special toxic substance to inhibit other kinds of microbes from increasing. Some of these substances can actually kill other microbes. A derivative of this special material is used to make antibiotics. This was a great discovery in modern medicine. There are many other products in everyday use that result from the work of microbes. Microbes and their enzymes are responsible for the production of vinegar (acetic acid), sauerkraut, soy sauce and miso, pickles, and other fermented foods. As I have already written, the human body carries billions of microbes, mainly in the large intestines, which help us clean the intestines and synthesize nutrients such as the B-vitamins.

What Really Causes Disease?

Now we can understand that microbes do not have to be feared, as you will recall from my remarks about Pettenkopfel and the cholera bacteria. What did Pettenkopfel's bold action teach us? In my opinion, it shows us that if we have a strong immune system, merely being exposed to bacteria cannot harm us.

After the work of Pasteur and Koch, microscopic research went on to discover many different kinds of bacteria and show how they were responsible for various diseases. While this research has contributed to the saving of countless lives, entirely too much emphasis was later placed on bacteria. In disease, microbes are only one side of the story; the other side is the body's immune system whose job it is to recognize and rid the body of any such harmful invaders. We always need to consider these two sides to understand the cause of diseases.

If we only look at the one side, we cannot effectively cure disease. Pasteur himself, for example, was stricken with a paralysis in one hemisphere of the body at the age of forty-six. There was no explanation at the time for the cause of his illness. Basically, causes have to do with the foods a person eats and how these foods affect blood chemistry, the immune system, and the various organs and systems of the body. If we could understand how certain foods support and others weaken the immune system, there could be a revolution in medicine.

Chapter 11

Life Units

Humans Are One

All human life is one. Beginning with our earliest ancestors and continuing through offspring, brothers, sisters, cousins, and so on, each human body is a single link in a potentially infinite chain. Since life first appeared on the earth this chain has never been severed; many branches separate into twos, tens, hundreds, and so on. When these branches connect and separate and connect again repeatedly, we call it intermarriage.

After a billion years these branches have increased into the billions, but the chain that binds them together – many different people and races, all human species – is just one.

Each link of the chain is an individual; what connects each link with all the others are the genes, located inside our body cells. Genes reproduce by duplication, creating exactly the same cells and the same genes. The special cells that connect the parents to their offspring are called the reproductive germ cells, namely, the father's sperm cell and the mother's egg cell, or ovum. Inside each reproductive germ are one-half of the father's genes and one-half of the mother's. These are the most important genes, carrying the characteristics of each individual.

The Mysterious Fertilized Egg

When the sperm and the egg combine, the two cells with their respective genes fuse with each other perfectly and become one cell and one set of genes. This cell is called the fertilized egg. Nothing in the world is more mysterious than this fertilized egg. The genes carry memory of the parents' body shape, size, structure, skin coloring, and hair as well as the inner functions and whole processes of construction. But the genes hold earlier memory, too, of the grandparents and great-grandparents, and further back to one billion years ago. For the father's body received two sets of genes, each of which is one-half of the genes of each of the grandparents, and the same for the mother. The grandparents, in turn, were recipients of two sets of genes which originated in the four great-grandparents, and so on back.

Genes and Evolution

Genes rarely make mistakes; generally, they exactly realize their encoded memory. We are fortunate that abnormal babies and sudden mutations seldom occur. But on the other hand, if genes were inflexibly resistant to change, then we would have no evolution. Rodents are always rodents, but this is actually not always the case.

To be exact, genes are always changing, but slowly. We hardly ever see such small changes, but with many generations repeating small changes, finally there can be a big change. Single-celled living organisms became double- and then multiple-celled, and further development resulted in human life. Scientists speculate that the fetus within its mother's body re-enacts this one-billion-year-old evolutionary process. As you can see, it is the genes that realize this scheduled plan.

In the mother's body the fertilized egg divides in two to make two cells which are exactly the same as the original. These two also divide and become four, but the genes remain the same as they were in the original fertilized egg. By the time three weeks have passed this division of the cells has resulted in a fetus (called an

Figure 7. Human Evolution Movie

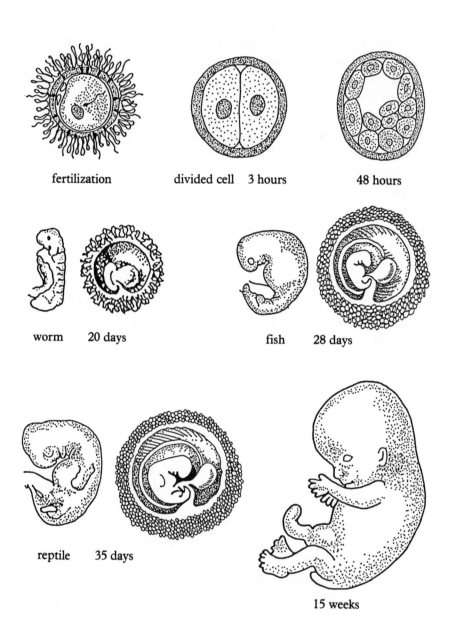

fertilization   divided cell   3 hours   48 hours

worm   20 days   fish   28 days

reptile   35 days

15 weeks

embryo) that looks like a worm or some kind of sea larva. Inside the fetus specific cells begin to form specific parts and organs of the body. These parts and their cells are constructed of various materials, but still in each cell the genes are the same. At four weeks we have something that looks like a fish; at six weeks it resembles a four-legged animal with tail and harelips. At this stage the human fetus appears little different from that of other mammals, but it then develops further. The harelips combine into one, the tail disappears, and finally, after around nine months, the fetus emerges as a brand new human baby.

During all of this time while the fetus develops its bone, muscle, skin, brain, and other organs of various cell tissues, the genes within each and every cell are exactly the same – just different parts of them are activated to create the various cells. That single fertilized egg cell has become an organism made up of some 2.5 trillion body cells, each with a copy of the original gene and its perfect memory.

A Billion Years in 280 Days

How much time was needed for the evolutionary process from our earliest ancestors to the present day is beyond our imagination. Therefore, here we will make a new movie called Human Evolution. In this movie let us assume that one second of time represents 10,000 years; one minute, 600,000 years; one hour, 36,000,000 years; twenty-eight hours, about 1,000,000,000 years.

This is the greatest drama that nature is producing, and it is the longest film ever made. As the movie starts, we can see only a tiny dot with our naked eye; we need a microscope to see a fertilized egg, which is just a single cell with the genetic memory of a billion years. We have to wait about three hours for the single cell to double itself; in the mother's body this occurs twenty-four hours after fertilization, or about 900 million years ago on the evolutionary scale. It seems that competition starts as soon as there are two cells and increases as the number of cells multiply. This competition is needed because otherwise cells would increase endlessly.

We then wait another three hours – forty-eight hours of mother's time – for the double cells to increase to sixteen. On the evolutionary scale this happened about 800 million years ago.

Another three hours go by and now the cells have increased to hundreds. This takes about seven days in mother's time, the stage of about 700 million years ago.

About fourteen hours from the beginning of our movie, the cells have multiplied into the hundreds of thousands. The embryo now resembles a worm. This is about twenty days after fertilization, so this stage was reached about 500 million years ago. Soon the embryo will look like a fish.

After about twenty-one hours of movie time, our embryo resembles an amphibian or reptile. This occurred probably 300 million years ago when our ancestors first came up onto land. Already some plants had crept onto the land, and these plants became the main food of our ancestors. Many varieties of plants and animals developed. In mother's time this happens at about four weeks. Now the growth process is accelerating.

After twenty-five hours of the movie, that is, about 100 million years ago, our ancestors still have tails and harelips. They look like small primitive rodents and are always hiding in holes or behind plants, running away from predators. Huge reptilian dinosaurs and other animals are attacking our ancestors on land and from the sky. But the weather and the composition of the air changed so that huge old plants disappeared and new ones producing seeds, grains, and nuts appeared. This time frame corresponds to about fifteen weeks after conception, mother's time.

Twenty-seven hours and forty-five minutes after starting our movie – ten million years ago – our ancestors have lost their tails and harelips and are standing and walking. They now look like monkeys or apes. Today this stage occurs at about thirty weeks following conception.

By now the huge reptiles have already become extinct and our ancestors have become strong and hardy animals. They can hold stones in their hands to protect against other animals.

Although they are increasing rapidly, their total numbers are still very small. They seem to have no special rules regarding sex, and they repeatedly intermarry. In the last five seconds of the movie – about 50,000 years ago – they have greatly increased. Many of them have separated from their brothers and cousins, left their native areas, and migrated throughout the world. The shape of the face, the color of the skin, hair, and eyes, and other small changes began at this time.

In the last second of the movie – 10,000 years ago – they are cultivating their foods and raising animals for meat and milk. They are now increasing in larger and larger numbers. They build large cities and some of them are always at war. In spite of this they still manage to increase. They take over all the territories which had belonged to the wild animals and construct the huge human empire. The last scene is all too short and disappointing, but it is true that the human evolutionary process takes such a long time.

A billion years of history have been seen in the space of a few minutes; the first cell developed into 2.5 trillion cells in the baby's body in just about 280 days. It is amazing that our genes can remember all of this process, rarely making a mistake. Please pay special attention to this good memory. It is crucially important for understanding life, healing power, and nature itself.

Acquired Characteristics and Genes

Research in this field has been carried out by a number of brilliant scientists; the most important part we owe to Charles Darwin, but other important names should not be overlooked. Immediately prior to Darwin's time there was Rudolf Virchow (1821-1902), who formulated the "cells from cells" theory (cells make new cells by duplicating themselves, thereby increasing). Louis Pasteur wrote, "Every living thing comes from a living thing;

all life is connected." Gregor Mendel (1822-1884) studied peas and discovered the laws governing heredity. August Weismann (1834-1914), considered to be the founder of modern genetics, stated that genes never change; genes from both parents just combine to form new life.

Both Darwin and Mendel faced much opposition in their time, for their theories were revolutionary. In the twentieth century both Mendel's Law and Weismann's theories were accepted by the scientific world and thereafter became the bases of all research on heredity. But these laws were not perfect, for if genes never change, we have no evolution.

In the last few decades a lot of new research has been done. Now almost everyone believes that acquired characteristics are absorbed into the genes. So Darwin was right. The environment in which we live, the foods we eat, the diseases we contract, our physical activity and thinking – everything becomes one part of our genes. These new memories may be weak at first, but through frequent repetition over a long period of time, the memory becomes stronger and the body slowly changes as a result.

Many Different Groups of Cells

We have many, many cells in our bodies, more than we can count; as an estimate, a baby has about 2.5 trillion cells while the adult body has around 75 trillion cells, each with the same genes inside. These tiny cells belong to larger groups, each of which forms an organ, muscle, or some other part of the body. Some of these groups contain thousands, some millions, of cells. The borders between these groups are well-defined, and the groupings may be seen as little kingdoms.

Cells are the smallest living units of the body, each separate from one other. To give a clearer image of this individualism, we can borrow from the old idea of "homunculus," meaning the little man. About two hundred years ago the developed scientific theory of heredity was that in the sperm the little man was a living being.

This could grow to a baby in a woman's womb. Of course, this is a primitive idea, but not so far-fetched. New research has determined that the genetic code, the DNA of both the mother and the father, contributes to the functioning of the baby. This is similar to the little man, only the image of a little man is changed to the image of the DNA code. The important point is that inside the cell the genes hold the memory of the whole body, copied exactly from the fertilized egg. We can imagine the body as a great empire of 75 trillion homunculi.

A Perfect Democracy

The cells are like the body's citizens, grouping together to form tissues that are like independent countries. Many tissues form organs and glands, kingdoms of many countries, which are all united under a great empire called the body. The citizens of each country or kingdom have various functions and structure, all requiring special nutrition; for example, bone needs more calcium and phosphorous, while the brain takes more sugar than the other organs.

But everything is provided by one source: blood, and nothing else. The average lifespan of each citizen differs widely; tissues of the stomach wall live for a day; white blood cells for about a month; some muscle and bone tissue cells for several years; and nerve cells for more than a hundred years.

Among the body cells, the body defines soldiers. The white blood cells are unique. They are completely independent and can move freely anywhere. In their structure and activity, they bear the most resemblance to bacteria or amoebas. They are working with a perfect information system. Red blood globules are called red blood cells, but actually these are not cells. They have no nucleus and no genetic code. They are just for carrying oxygen and a few other functions.

We know that the brain, which contains a vast number of cells – some 150 billion of them – controls all the united kingdoms, but who controls the brain? No one. There is no king or government to rule these 150 billion citizens of the brain. All of them are equal workers, performing as a perfect team. This is possible because each cell knows the entire body through the gene pool and because all the genes derive from one original set. Not only the brain cells, but all the body cells know the entire body. This is probably the origin of our intuition, or the so-called sixth sense. Even if we don't know something by thinking, we can sense it through the memory and information provided through the genes. This is important in emergencies, sometimes appearing as a super power. Thus, the genes are like the brain of each body cell.

The Origin of Healing Power

New research on the immune system has shown that lymphocytes can multiply independently if they are needed to fight against the microbes that are causing a specific disease. They can clone themselves, one becoming two, two four, four eight and so on. The source of this ability remains a mystery, but the genes inside these cells are encoded strongly with the knowledge of the fertilized egg.

The most important healing ability comes from cell duplication. In a group of tuberculosis patients, x-rays showed such severely damaged lungs that no hope of recovery was offered. Still, some patients did recover, and subsequent radiographs revealed that the recovery was complete, with no trace of the disease. Many people would claim that this is a mystery, but our cells can do mysterious things. If some healthy cells remain, they can duplicate and generate new cells where diseased cells were destroyed. Their power is very similar to that of the fertilized egg. It has been claimed that all our organs have this power; the liver especially excels in this ability of self-recovery. However, brain cells have no ability to reproduce; once they die, there is no recovery of normal functioning.

In regard to injuries, we notice that when we cut our skin, although it often looks very bad, we almost always recover nicely. Skin cells have a good ability of reproduction, especially in small children due to their better metabolism. For them, scars can be slight, and when they reach the age of fifteen to twenty the scars often have disappeared altogether.

If we lose a finger or a hand or any other limb, it will not grow back, as the original cells needed for reproduction have been used. Cells from another group cannot work like the fertilized egg cell. If we lose a muscle, recovery depends on the severity of the injury. If the cut is deep, we may lose the cells of the "master copies," in which case we will not have a perfect recovery; but if the master copies remain intact, they can duplicate. Broken bones also recover nicely provided they are properly set; if so, they will combine neatly, just as they were prior to injury. Even if some bone has been lost, there can be regeneration if the bone membrane has not been damaged. In this case we may not have a success rate of 100 percent, but can expect about 70 to 80 percent recovery.

These examples demonstrate the body's ability to heal itself; however, this ability is much affected by the nutrition provided through the blood. The body's healing power comes mainly from cell metabolism, the process of destroying old cells and rebuilding new ones being conducted by the gene's memory.

For example, in the case of a broken bone, if the blood does not contain enough calcium, recovery will occur, but more slowly. If the calcium level is too high, the excess calcium may form deposits in the broken areas, causing the healed bones to be abnormally large in size or malformed. In the case of a skin cut, the recovery will be slow if there is not enough protein in the blood; too much protein, on the other hand, will cause big scars which may never disappear.

How the Cells Live

Once more, think about the image of the little man for each body cell. They do not look like human bodies, but they are living independently, except for receiving nutrition and oxygen from the blood and special instructions from the brain through circulating hormones in the blood. The cell knows what kind of nutrients it needs and what it doesn't need. It takes the exact quantity of what it needs and no more.

Cells take carbohyrates and oxygen and produce heat to maintain the body's temperature and activities. They take protein and reproduce more cells. The cells work together to facilitate all kinds of bodily functions and activities. The health of the cells is the health of the body; disease of the cells is disease of the body, as Rudolf Virchow discussed.

Cells are divided by membranes. Some materials pass through these membranes and other materials are rejected, depending on necessity. For example, the proportion of sodium and potassium in the fluids which are inside and outside of the cells is crucially important for the cell's health and function. Cellular fluid should be high in potassium and low in sodium while the fluids outside the cells, blood and lymph, contain much sodium. The cell membrane controls these amounts very strictly by the functions of what are often called the sodium pump and the potassium pump; the cells simply do not accept any excess.

Small and Sensitive

Cells are so tiny (about one-one millionth of a meter), invisible to the naked eye, but their activities, functions, and sensitivities are just amazing. These functions indicate that cells not only have perfect memory of the whole body but also have memory of many kinds of materials which are circulating in the blood. Where such memory is kept is a big question. Some scholars say that the cell keeps the entire memory in its RNA (ribonucleic acid), one form of genetic code. If this is so, then the RNA would be the brain of the cell and would control all cellular functions.

In any case, the environment of the cells and the quality of the blood and lymph should be kept at an optimal state. For this purpose, many organs are working together all the time. The liver, kidneys, lungs, intestines, and many endocrine glands regulate the composition of blood by the needs of the cells. This is called blood homeostasis. Cells are so sensitive that the smallest change in blood quality can cause cellular activity to slow down or stop. It can even cause the death of the cell.

Still, each organ has a certain capacity to regulate. Eating a large amount of nutritionally unbalanced food can change the quality of the blood and disturb the organ's normal function of regulation. Food should be chosen very carefully.

One more very important and influential factor for healthy cells is any synthetic or even natural chemical or drug – whether medicinal, recreational, in the form of a food additive, or any other kind. All such unfamiliar foreign substances disturb the normal functioning of organs and cells.

Please remember that the purpose of our eating is to feed 75 trillion homunculi, the body cells.

Chapter 12

The Immune System

The Body is a Battlefield

In Chapter 10 we saw that microbes are everywhere – in the air, in water, in foods, and in our body. They live on the surface of the skin always ready to attack us; even if we took ten showers a day we could not wash them away completely. They continue to increase and attack, always looking for a good place and the nutrition to grow. Therefore the inside of our body is the battlefield of a never-ending war. It is said that about four different microbes invade a person's body every day. That means fifteen hundred invasions a year, about one hundred thousand in a lifetime of seventy years. It is crucial that we never lose even one of these battles; if we do, it can be fatal.

The whole body is covered by a strong barrier of skin. Microbes, water, or many kinds of chemicals cannot penetrate this barrier. The body excretes sebum (oil) and sweat which contain a variety of chemical agents such as oleic acid, lactic acid, and salt that are capable of intercepting and destroying harmful microbes. Mucous membranes secrete tears and are protected by saliva and mucous, which also contains a special enzyme, lysozyme, and other substances to kill microorganisms and wash them away, thus keeping the surface clean.

The blood and tissue fluids contain many kinds of protective substances such as spermime, properdin, and defensin to kill microbes. But these are prepared defense mechanisms and have no special reaction against attacks from aggressive microbes.

Defense Forces

The most important defense soldiers of the body are the white blood cells, the leukocytes. They are classified as phagocytes and lymphocytes. Phagocytes are eating-cells (feeding or scavenger cells) which are always patrolling the whole body in search of any foreign invaders. If they find enemies, the phagocytes engulf them and send out a chemical warning to other friendly soldiers. Macrophages, microphages, and granulocytes are examples of this type of white blood cell.

Other kinds of defense soldiers are the white blood cells called lymphocytes. All white blood cells probably originated in the bone marrow, but they receive special training from different organs. The stem cells, immature cells from bone marrow, migrate to the thymus gland and become T-cells. Then they go back into the bloodstream and many of them go into the lymphoid organs.

Now understood to be one of the most important organs for the immune system, the thymus gland gives special training for the stem cells. During the hard training many weak cells die. Only about 5 percent graduate from this military school and become defense officers, T-cells. Helper T-cells, killer T-cells, suppressor T-cells are all such kind of cells. In the case of AIDS, the number of helper T-cells is decreased significantly.

The stem cells which receive special training from intestinal mucous membrane tissue, lymph nodes, liver, or spleen become B-cells. Their special abilities are that they produce antibodies and that they are monoclonal, which means that they can multiply quickly from one to two, two to four, four to eight, and so on. These are plasma cells. Plasma cells produce antibodies.

Weapons

Antibodies are the most powerful weapons against the attack of microbes or any antigen, a foreign substance which invades the body. B-cells produce specific antibodies to each of many various antigens, for the body needs innumerable numbers of various antibodies. Actually, it is said that the body is capable of producing and maintaining one million or more different antibodies.

Once the antibodies have been made and the battle is over, the body liquidates all but two thousand or so of each kind of antibody which form the memory pool. If the body receives a second attack from the same antigen, the antibodies multiply suddenly into the millions and immediately attack. Therefore, the body almost never succumbs to the same antigen during its lifetime. This ability is called immunity, or we say that the body is immune to a specific disease.

The antibodies are very important weapons in the body's defense system, but their production is rather slow – from one to three months. If the virus settles inside the body cells, the antibodies, once produced, cannot find the virus and do not attack the body cells. But, before antibodies have been made or the white blood cells can react to a viral attack, the body produces antiviral substances called interferons. These inhibitors of viral multiplication are also anticancer substances and are most important in the early stages of viral diseases.

Interferons are effective for many kinds of viruses and can be cultivated in other human cells. However, they are difficult to inject into a patient's body because the body often reacts to the injected interferon as a foreign substance, and shock or other troubles result. So, research advanced to the next step. A special material was discovered from an extract of shiitake mushroom which stimulates body cells to produce more interferons. This special material, called an interferon inducer, can be injected or given orally in liquid form. Other foods also contain this substance. This is one of the most promising developments in the prevention of viral diseases and cancer.

Complement factors which are maintained in the tissue fluids are always circulating in the blood. These tiny particles are also important weapons for fighting microorganisms. They are activated by the antigen-antibody reaction and start to work. The complement factors can increase the blood flow to the battlesite and can call forth more white blood cells. White blood cells are able to pass through the walls of blood vessels or lymph vessels, but complement factors make such passage easier. Also, they attach themselves to the bodies of microbes and cause the microbes to be readily ingested by macrophages.

Systematic Defense

The lymphatic system is a network of lymph vessels throughout the whole body. From this network small vessels emerge, pass to a neighboring branch, become larger and larger, and finally connect the thoracic duct with blood vessels. The prime purpose of this system is the draining of tissue fluid and returning protein to the bloodstream, but it is also very important for the the tranportation of the body's defenses. In the normal condition, red blood cells are not allowed to enter this system, probably because they would disturb the smooth flow of traffic (although the ends of the lymphatic system are connected with the blood vessels). The entire system fills up with lymphatic fluid which is composed mainly of salt water and certain other components.

The lymphatic system has many lymph nodes, the forts and fortresses that serve as the bases of the defense network. Hundreds of them are strung along the lymph vessels and many are located at the intersections and joints of the branches.

Local Battle

If the front line of defense, the skin, is broken and microbes penetrate under it to attack unarmed body cells and thus take the cells' nutrition, the destroyed cells release substances which enter the blood and lymph system. This is the chemical sign of alarm to local defense soldiers which are always patrolling everywhere. Blood permeates the broken site to repair it and to bring more white blood cells.

Macrophages start eating the invaders. Helper T-cells send a full-scale alarm to the various units of the body's defense system and also direct troop operations. With this, alarm troops of soldiers are mobilized. Much blood comes to the battlesite and the blood vessels swell up. The affected area becomes red and hot because blood brings heat from the interior of the body. Swollen tissues give pressure to sensory nerves and one feels pain. This is an inflammation, just a small local battle.

If the invaders are powerful, they multiply and spread over a wider area. Then, more defense troops arrive and the battle becomes more severe. If the enemies are defeated, the white blood cells clean the dead bodies and damaged cells are carried out by the blood. The wound goes into the healing process. In the case of a larger battle, if the damage from both sides is too large and the blood cannot clean everything readily, the body pushes out needless substances and forms an abscess and pus to clean the area quickly.

Before the local battle is expanded and in order to avoid body cell damage, the white cells try to lead the invaders into the lymph vessels. Then, the invaders ride on the lymph stream and easily advance to the local lymph nodes, heavily armed defense forts with plenty of soldiers – T-cells, B-cells, plasma-cells, and antibodies waiting to fight. Here, filtering tissue checks everything that comes in and detains foreign invaders, and white blood cells kill them. This is also the site where the B-cells multiply and produce antibodies. Often the nodes swell because of the increased white blood cells and antibodies and because the amount of blood increases in the lymph tissue capillaries to reinforce friendly soldiers.

Full-scale War
The phagocytes react to bacterial toxins, produce interleukin-1,

and activate the lymphocytes and the whole immune system. As the interleukin-1 increases in the blood it reaches the brain and the brain orders the hypothalamus to produce fever. From this regulation center and through the autonomic nervous system and hormonal controls, all the body cells know that a full-scale war is being waged.

The body cells become active and produce more heat in order to kill the invading enemies. At the very least, heat inhibits microbial activity and multiplication. The human body's enzymes are most active between the temperatures of 102°F and 104°F. All organs become more active: the heart beats more and sends more blood, the liver destroys more protein, the kidneys excrete more waste products, and so on. On the other hand, the consumption of nutrients increases significantly and the body loses weight. If the body's defense forces lose a local battle, the invaders advance to the next lymph node. However, this kind of war may occur anywhere in the body and is not limited to the lymph nodes only.

The last defense bases are the large lymph nodes of the groin, neck, or armpits – several sets are located in each of these areas. This struggle is the peak of the war. The body uses its full force, taking reserves from the spleen and other lymphoid tissues. The nodes swell up, sometimes to a huge size. Once this defense fortress has been penetrated, the enemies invade the internal organs and attack. This is the worst thing that can happen, for the organs, unlike the lymph system, are not protected with such a battery of armed forces.

Fortunately, however, microbes are not always powerful such as those of the bubonic plague. Most of the wars are smaller. Without our awareness or any uncomfortable feeling, many wars end silently. If we check carefully, many people have one or more swollen lymph nodes. This is not considered a dangerous situation. Also, note that the lymph nodes remain swollen for a while after the war has subsided.

Other Lymphoid Organs

The spleen is the largest organ containing lymphoid tissue. This tissue filters out foreign invaders and detains or kills them in the same way as the lymph nodes, but this is not for main battles. This is comparable to a quartermaster storing reserve force weapons (antibodies) and much blood, and providing training for the B-cells.

Formerly, adenoids and tonsils were thought to be needless glands and were often removed surgically. But now, the newer understanding is that these glands are like a checking station, constructed with lymphoid tissue and located at the entrance of the digestive tract and air tube. They are also armed with many lymphocytes which check out invaders and detain as many as possible so they may be killed. The adenoids and tonsils often receive a counter-attack from the enemies and swell up. But, as long as the battle is confined to these glands, the body is considered to be safe.

The appendix is also thought of as useless vestigial tissue, but this structure is also lymphoid tissue and heavily armed with forces and weapons. The exact function is not understood well, but at least it is not needless tissue because it plays an important role in protecting the body from harmful microbes.

Actually, the immune system of the body is much more complicated. Here, I have tried to outline the body's perfect defense mechanism so you can understand its role in health and disease. It is said that the immune system is the most sophisticated system in the human body next to the brain, for it is dealing with the problem of life or death.

The Origin of the Immune System

Scholars say that the Pacific Ocean is the oldest sea on the earth. When our ancestors lived in the ocean, our whole world was peaceful, as the modern name of this ocean suggests. But after these microorganisms increased and developed into multi-celled living things which evolved in many different ways, some species began to eat others. Now we had to fight, we had to protect ourselves; otherwise, we could be eaten. Single-celled microbes often invaded our body, which had to develop a defense system for survival. This was the origin of our immune system. As we developed, so did our immune system. "We" or "our" refer to our ancestors, but their genes were the same as ours.

Probably for 900 million years or more, trillions of battles and wars have been ceaselessly fought in our bodies. Of course, many of our brothers and sisters failed to survive these wars which have always been crucial events in our history. But live or die, we could not have afforded to lose a single war. Some developed defense mechanisms in their bodies and survived. The experience of battle became the gene's memory and made for stronger offspring. As the body evolved, the immune system developed and finally the modern human body and immune system was completed.

Never-Defeated Champions

Since the beginning, microbes have always been with us. They mutate and take many forms, but they all came from the same ancestors. They are very small and their structures have remained extremely simple. Microbes have had no great evolution and completely new microbes have never emerged.

Since billions and trillions of wars have been fought in the body, the genes must have all these in their memory. So, why do some people lose this defense? The reason is immune system deterioration.

Think about the last one thousand years. Our ancestors have had so many plagues and epidemics which attacked them repeatedly – the Black Death, cholera, malaria, smallpox, tuberculosis, and many others. Each time so many, from 10 to 40 percent or more of those infected, died. But still we are here. Thus, we are the descendants of the strongest, the never-defeated champions.

New Disease or Old?

Many people are afraid that AIDS is a new disease and that it will wipe us all out. This is not true, for we hardly ever have a completely new disease. Again, I want to illustrate with historical events. Take syphilis, for example, since at the time of its eruption this was thought to be a new disease. The story goes as follows.

In 1494 A.D. the French King Charles VIII started the Italian War by invading Naples. The first cases of syphilis were recorded at this time. As always happens under the conditions of war, the soldiers on both sides were very undisciplined. There was a lot of raping and ravaging of women – anyplace, anytime, and with all kinds of women. A new epidemic broke out and spread as a result of the soliders' conduct – a very unexpected result of the war. The Italian people blamed the French, calling the disease the "French Disease," while the French, of course, referred to it as the "Italian or Neapolitan disease." Since the time of Fracastoro's famous poem, most people have accepted the Italian version.

In 1492, just prior to the Italian War, Christopher Columbus arrived in the Caribbean Islands, thinking that they were "Gipango" (the mythical Gold Islands of Japan). In March of the following year he returned to Europe, disembarking in Portugal. Some scholars argue that Columbus's crew brought syphilis back with them from the New World; however, no records exist indicating that the disease was contracted either by the sailors or by the Native Americans they had met in the course of their explorations.

Another argument against this theory is that people still used foot or horseback as their principal means of transportation at that time. It seems highly unlikely that in such a short time syphilis could have spread from Spain to Naples. It appears that Columbus did have syphilis when he returned from his third voyage in 1504. The condition of his whole body was described at that time as being dropsical, a term suited for syphilis. If the above argument disproving the origin of syphilis from the New World is correct, then syphilis is not a new disease. Even apart from the issue of origin, the fact remains that many people exposed to syphilis did not contract it, while others did; furthermore, some recovered without any treatment whatsoever. Also, records show that women were more resistant to this disease.

New research has suggested that the early theories as to the origin of syphilis are incorrect. This realization opened up first as a result of the study of yaws, an old disease prevalent in tropical countries, not transmitted sexually. The yaws bacteria is very similar to the syphilis bacteria and belongs to the same family; this theory suggested that the bacteria mutates, goes into the body from the sexual organs, and creates symptoms of syphilis. This idea was not widely accepted, however, due to the lack of further evidence.

Other research came from some ancient records. More than four thousand years ago the Chinese had written about a genital disease quite similar to syphilis, and ancient Greek and Roman documents also mentioned this. Anthropological studies have found ancient skeletons whose bones have unique marks of the syphilis infection. Old records show that many crusade warriors contracted leprosy, but this was really syphilis. After world trading increased in the sixteenth century, many people ate imported foods and worsened their health condition. The disease spread all over the world.

The syphilis bacteria, once it enters the bloodstream and spreads, will destroy any part of the body, any of the organs, and in particular the brain. Children often had congenital syphilis which they contracted from an infected mother. Syphilis is a sexually transmitted disease and has always had a strong connection with promiscuity.

It is worthy of notice that syphilis has had a preference for royal families, nobility, politicians, and the rich over the peasants and ordinary citizens. The political decline of the dominance of the Valois in France and of the Ottoman in Turkey is directly related to the prevalence of this disease, for one of its effects is the generation of weakened and unhealthy offspring. King Edward VI and Queen Mary are, among others, examples of famous people who were known to be victims of syphilis.

For the last five hundred years, syphilis has been widespread and one of the most formidable diseases. In the early twentieth century the famous pioneer of modern chemotherapy and hematology, Paul Ehrlich, made a drug called salvarsan with an organic compound containing arsenic that would kill the syphilis bacteria in a patient's body. After 606 trials he finally succeeded in making the first effective drug to control syphilis. He was respected like a savior.

But after about twenty years of wide use, bacteria developed resistance to salvarsan and it became less effective. Many sulfa drugs were made to take its place but again, after about twenty years, these became less effective. Then, penicillin came into practical use. This organic compound was so effective that often just one injection killed all the syphilis bacteria in the body. But again new strains have recently developed and penicillin and other antibiotics have lost their effectiveness. A series of multiple antibiotic injections has been used, but it is still a difficult disease to treat.

In 1973, CAT (computerized axial tomography) scanners began to be used in medical examinations. This device has brought dramatic developments in medical diagnosis. In scanning ancient Egyptian and Peruvian mummies, clear evidence of disease in the ancient human body has been found. Some of the skeletons reveal the unique lesions of syphilis. This anthropological evidence leads us to the new understanding that human disease has not changed essentially since the earliest of times.

Is AIDS Really New?

Now let's apply the lessons of syphilis to our modern-day concern with AIDS. As I have already shown, AIDS is probably not a new disease; the infections accompanying AIDS are certainly well known.

A hundred years ago Moriz Kaposi found and reported a special kind of skin tumor, and in 1909 Carlos Chagas observed a disease now known as PCP (*Pneumocystis carinii* pneumonia) caused by a generally harmless protozoa.[1] Since that time, similar diseases have often been reported in Africa, Europe, and the United States that seem to fit the description of diseases associated with AIDS.

Neither are the other opportunistic infections commonly associated with AIDS entirely new. Cytomegalovirus is the most common cause of death among AIDS patients, but before AIDS was identified it was known as one of many very common and usually harmless germs. Another is EBV (Epstein-Barr virus) which is known to cause mononucleosis, the "kissing disease" that is very common but seldom fatal. *Candida albicans,* the yeast infection also known as thrush, is, according to Dr. Frederick Siegal, "part of the normal 'flora' of the body's microbial garden. It is one of the countless germs that live on or in us, causing no disease but rather contributing in various ways to our well-being by helping to digest our food and providing us with vitamins."[2]

These are just a few of the many relatively harmless or even beneficial microscopic organisms that are part of the delicate balance of our life and biosphere. When the immune system is weakened by the use of drugs, antibiotics, and the excessive and habitual consumption of certain foods, this balance is thrown off and many diseases can result. In other words, people are dying of illnesses caused by microbes that are otherwise practically harmless.

Weakened Immune System

AIDS is a disease characterized by the suppression of the immune system (immuno-suppressive). The number of helper T-cells has decreased dramatically. Taking advantage of this immuno-suppressed condition, other microbes launch an attack in the same patient. This combining of forces has been a rather recent discovery.

The culprit responsible for AIDS has been identified as the virus HTLV-HIV, although this connection has not yet been absolutely determined. There is also some doubt as to whether the HTLV-III virus belongs to the same species as the virus HTLV-I, the virus which causes leukemia and lymphoma (cancers of the blood and lymphatic system). HTLV-III cannot cause leukemia or tumors, but mainly attacks helper T-cells and brain cells. There is no question that HTLV-I has been around for a long time.

The diseases assigned to the HTLV-I virus are found chiefly in southwestern Japan, the Caribbean Islands, and to a lesser extent in tropical Africa and the southeastern United States. The HTLV-I cancer is a very rare but contagious disease, considered to have been in southern Japan for the past three hundred years. One hypothesis for this connection is that the Portuguese carried HTLV-I to Japan and the Carribean Islands with their African slaves or in monkeys in the sixteenth century. But this cannot explain why this virus did not spread in the Pacific Islands and elsewhere. In my opinion, the disease accompanied the cultivation of sugar. After the Japanese learned to grow sugar cane, it was cultivated for about three hundred years only in this area. The people in this region, with their traditionally high fish intake, contracted the disease. The same picture emerges in the Caribbean. Later on, some who lived in Florida were infected.

Japanese doctors discovered positive reactions to antibodies of HTLV-I among the residents of these sugar-producing areas; they also found similar results in many people who lived on the main island and among the Ainu (who live only on Hokkaido Island in the northeast of Japan), but in these cases the people tested never actually came down with the disease. This means that, although the virus had spread throughout all of Japan, it had not caused an outbreak of disease except in the southernmost areas.

Now that sugar is everywhere, it is possible that the disease will spread elsewhere, but this has not yet happened.

It has been estimated that the total number of those who suffer from this leukemia/lymphoma is only about two thousand worldwide. Also, like other cancers, it is a slow-growing disease, taking from ten to twenty years to develop. For these reasons there is not that much concern about the disease; however, researchers are greatly interested in it because of the virus. The point at issue is whether a virus can cause cancer.

Immunity Lost

The big fear surrounding AIDS is largely the result of a lack of understanding as to what factors weaken the immune system in the first place, allowing this disease to render the victim practically defenseless in the face of the relatively harmless microbes found in his environment.

Let us look at measles and chicken pox. Everyone infected by these viruses will acquire immunity from them and after recovery be free of them for the remainder of their lives. It is rare for anyone who has had these diseases to suffer a recurrence. This is a well-known fact. Almost 100 percent of exposed subjects are infected but the majority recover fully. This also means that our ancestors had experience with these diseases and we developed genetic resistance, as opposed to a less common disease such as rabies, which is still quite dangerous. Our ancestors never won the fight against that virus.

However, despite our common immunity against measles following recovery, many years later some people will contract multiple sclerosis (MS), a disease that causes irreversible damage to the nerves. New research has indicated that MS is caused by an attack of the measles virus followed by a secondary attack of the mumps, rubella, or flu virus. An even more terrible disease, subacute sclerosingencephalopathy, which causes brain damage, is considered to be completely fatal. Most cases are found in boys around the age of fifteen. Researchers suspected some kind of a lentivirus as the culprit here, but electron microscopy revealed that this virus was none other than the measles virus. Ten years earlier these boys either had had the measles or had been vaccinated for them, and later the same virus attacked again, fatally. I think this was caused by acute deterioration of the body's immune system, brought on by excess consumption of sugars and chemicals. The reason behind my thinking is explained in Chapter 14.

Genetic Memory

Tuberculosis is an airborne bacteria to which probably everyone at some time or another is exposed. But even when TB reached its peak (around the middle of the nineteenth century) less than 20 percent of the American and European populations became infected. The highest mortality rates were reported in Philadelphia in 1845: 618 per 100,000. The United States average was about 400 per 100,000 or 0.4 percent, which, compared with other plagues, is rather low. From this we can assume that our genes have had more experience in dealing with this disease.

The common cold is one of the most familiar diseases. It is said that its cause is a virus, but this is more complicated, as there are more than one hundred different strains of virus that can cause this disease. Nearly everyone gets a cold once or several times a year, so that in the last million years our ancestors had at least a million individual experiences of it. Our genes remember the cold as a disease rather easily handled. Since viruses are everywhere, almost everyone is exposed, but only a percentage are infected and the mortality rate is extremely low. The common cold is not even listed within the top fifteen in tables that provide death rates.

Probably viruses are microbes that had a later development, since they cannot live without host cells. As causative agents of disease they are relative latecomers. Viruses and the diseases they cause, including the AIDS virus, are less familiar to our bodies than bacterial diseases; our ancestors have had less experience with them. Still, the rate of those who are infected with AIDS, as compared against the great numbers of those who are exposed to it, is extremely low. This means that we have enough experience to beat this virus. The AIDS virus itself is not even as powerful as the viruses that cause hepatitis, polio, or measles.

Statistical research has shown that around 90 percent of those exposed to the HIV-I AIDS virus develop antibodies to the virus. This is proof enough that AIDS can be prevented, for if the body cannot produce antibodies it will never be capable of developing immunity. The remaining 10 percent have no ability to produce antibodies in spite of the fact that they have full-blown AIDS.

Recent Enemies

In the natural world many organic poisons exist, but over time we have developed ways to protect ourselves against them. All living things – animals, plants, microbes – are composed of organic materials, the same components that make up the matter of our body. For us, cleaning out organic matter is a relatively easy task. But new drugs, chemicals, and poor quality nutrients that disturb our genetic memory are recent enemies that our ancestors never experienced. Modern-day chemicals are new compounds artificially made by human beings. In the past all organic materials came from living organisms. But in recent years many so-called organic materials are synthesized artificially. Many of these are not suitable as human or animal food. Since these materials do not occur naturally in the body, they are all more or less toxic in their effects. Arsenic, for example, is a strong poison, but a small amount of organic arsenic exists as an essential mineral in our body. On the other hand, a small amount of inorganic arsenic can be fatal. Today, many chemical agents are used in medicines, food additives, insecticides, and many other products; these are not harmonious with our body.

One of the most commonly used chemicals on the market is aspirin, considered a most useful medicine. It relieves the pain of headache and arthritis; reduces heart attacks; lowers high fevers; induces restful sleep, etc. But now many adverse toxic side effects have been reported. Aspirin is known to be an irritant to the stomach and the intestines, where it causes mucosal erosion of the inside walls. The intestines can lose the ability to absorb iron, which can lead to anemia. Aspirin is also linked to asthma and Reye's Syndrome, a children's disease of viral origin which begins with the respiratory and digestive organs, leading to convulsions, swelling of the brain, and coma; it is a highly fatal disease. Aspirin can cause birth defects and low birth weight, factors that contribute to a high mortality rate among the newborn. Often severe reactions such as allergies, kidney damage, and other serious side-effects have been reported. These are acute reactions, but there are probably many other chronic reactions that will appear later on. We may be able to estimate how many cures have been attributed to aspirin, but we cannot estimate the negative effects.

Saccharin was also widely used, its popularity having begun as early as 1900. Since then it has been used in dietetic foods, in diet soft drinks, and, because it has no calories, as a recommended sugar substitute, especially for diabetics and the obese. For the same reason it was thought to be helpful in fighting tooth decay. Saccharin has been used freely for more than eighty years, but the government just recently prohibited its general use due to its potential cancer risk based on laboratory animal tests. As research develops, many long-used food additives and other chemicals formerly thought to be safe are found to have toxic effects and are gradually disappearing from the market. All chemicals repress the immune system. One of the roles of the white blood cells is to remove foreign matter from our systems. This essentially important defense force should not be wasted on such avoidable toxins.

Antibiotics

Many chemotherapeutic drugs have immuno-suppressive effects and are used widely for organ transplants as I have already reported. However, the most powerful and most widely used new antibiotics are not immuno-suppressive drugs. They are organic materials which with frequent use create the most powerful effects of immune suppression. Many antibiotics are now produced and they can kill almost any kind of bacteria. People have expected that all kinds of bacteria which cause disease can be eradicated.

Surely the antibiotics can kill bacteria, but what happens to the body's natural immune system? Probably the white blood cells won't need to work and will become lazy, or the body will reduce production of its defense forces. As a result, immune deficiency may appear. This kind of body deterioration is similar to muscles which atrophy if we don't use them. Many AIDS patients have had repeated antibiotic treatments for syphilis, gonorrhea, and other diseases before they have contracted AIDS.

I am suspicious of the widespread and increasing cases of AIDS in Haiti. In 1954, the Haitian government forced the entire population to receive penicillin therapy for curing and preventing yaws. The project was sponsored by the World Health Organization (WHO) and was the first attempt to try to eradicate a certain kind of infection. Almost 90 percent of the Haitians received this treatment. Yaws is a skin infection caused by bacteria very similar but not identical to syphilis and is commonly called pinta or raspberry disease. Yaws decreased dramatically, but other diseases are increasing quickly and now they are facing the problem of AIDS.

In African countries where the incidence of AIDS is high, antibiotics are over-the-counter drugs and anyone can buy them without a prescription. They have heard that the new medications are effective. Tourists are asked if they have any drugs because the Africans want to trade fruit or handicrafts for them.

The Cause of Viral Mutation

What causes viral mutation? We have to think one step further.

A virus is the smallest and most primitive living organism and can mutate very easily and cause different diseases. As a general rule, mutation and evolution are caused mainly by different environments and foods. For the virus, the host cell provides the environment and nutrition; therefore, in the natural world mutation does not occur so often. But in the modern human body, the body cells often receive chemical substances which our ancestors' cells never experienced. The change can be very small and only temporary, but for the virus this can be strong poison. But still they survive by mutating, and the mutations are able to resist the chemicals.

This process is the same for bacteria, which also develop new resistant strains. Then, clearly we are making new viruses or bacteria as we saw in the case of syphilis. Modern techniques produce more powerful medications and stimulate microbial mutations. This competition seems to have no end. From the point of view of the body's immune system, this is not a positive development but rather retrogression. Ironically, the new medications are producing the deterioration of our bodies. Not only chemicals, but also sugar and other refined foods, well-preserved foods, and all kinds of substances unfamiliar to the body's cells can contribute to the mutation of microbes.

Changing the Focus

Around the end of the nineteenth century, the medical world devoted much time and interest to the study of microbes as causative agents of disease. In reaction to this trend, one man stood out in his research, not of microbes but of the defense system of human and animal bodies. He was the discoverer of macrophages, white blood cells which move like amoebas and engulf bacteria in our bodies.

The man's name was Elie Metchnikoff, considered today as the founder of immunology. In 1904 he received the Nobel Prize in medicine for his research, an honor that surprised many people throughout the world, for Metchnikoff was not a physician, but a zoologist. His discovery is considered to be as significant as Louis Pasteur's work with disease-causing microbes and as van Leeuwenhoeh's discovery of bacteria in the seventeenth century.

Whereas microbial research developed rapidly, studies on the immune system proceeded at a slow pace. But today, since the outbreak of AIDS, research on the immune system has come to the fore as being more urgent than the study of causative agents.

If we could determine immune deterioration very early, then AIDS could be prevented and not only AIDS but also many infectious diseases; even cancer could become preventable. My dream is to reach this goal through some means of measuring the immune power of every person. It should be something as simple as taking a temperature or blood pressure. Both the healthy and the sick could be checked anytime.

Already some kind of measurement has been devised. There are tests available for counting the number of white blood cells, B-cells, and T-cells (including helper T-cells, suppressor T-cells, and others). But these cells constitute only one part of the immune system. Interferons, interleukins, hormones, antibody formations, as well as many other factors, all work together for a strong immune system. To calculate the effectiveness of each of these factors would be far too complicated, but there is another way. Liebig's "law of minimum" could be applied. The idea would be that the weakest factor would determine the effectiveness and power of all factors combined.

Immunity Score

Medical tests, innumerable and costly, are not practical for everyone. So here I want to offer six conditions of self-examination in order to help determine how your immune system is functioning. It will not work for sick people or for those taking prescribed medicine, but the majority of people in a normal health condition can get a rough idea. It is determined almost entirely by your feelings and observations of the surface of the body, and is very easy.

Condition 1: Your skin has a nice natural shine and is not too oily or too dry. There are no pimples or rashes and the color is clear, regardless of the pigment. You do not attract any insects such as fleas, ticks, mosquitos, or houseflies. Even if you get a bite or if you have a small cut, nothing more than a tiny inflammation occurs. In cold weather you may sometimes have some common cold-like symptoms, but no fever above 101°F, no headaches, not much coughing, and no other suffering. This condition means that the immune system is working properly; you are safe.

Condition 2: You sometimes have skin inflammations from small cuts or insect bites, but they go away without any treatment. Sometimes you have pimples or skin rashes, but they don't become serious skin trouble. A couple of times each winter you have a common cold, but it can be cured without any medication. This means your immune system is working at about 90 percent.

Condition 3: Even if you have skin trouble, inflammations, or infections, they go away with the use of common ointments or simple medications. You catch cold several times per year, but the fever does not exceed 103°F; there are no severe headaches, coughing, or body pain. The cold subsides with simple treatment within a few days. This means about 80 percent of your immune system is working.

Condition 4: You have long-lasting or frequent skin troubles such as pimples, rashes, flaky skin, or skin infections. Also, you often catch colds or flu and sometimes, but not always, need prescription drugs or antibiotics. This means your immune function is about 70 percent (30 percent down), and you are in a slightly dangerous condition for contracting AIDS or a serious infection.

Condition 5: You have *Candida*, eczema, psoriasis, or other serious skin disease inflammation, or an infection for which you frequently need antibiotics. You may be continually taking antibiotics to prevent infection. You have chronic respiratory system trouble such as bronchitis, bronchial asthma, or tuberculosis and are often treated with epinephrine or cortisone, streptomycin or viomycin. You catch colds in the summertime and they persist for a long time, and you repeat the same symptoms the following year. This means you have lost more than 40 percent of your immune ability. This is a dangerous state. Be careful in contact with AIDS patients.

Condition 6: You have had a sexually transmitted disease or other serious infectious disease and have had multiple-antibiotic treatments. Even if you feel fine right now, it is possible that you have lost about 50 percent of your immune function. If you are exposed to the AIDS virus, you could be infected very easily.

Chapter 13

The Harmony and Balance of the World

Life Everywhere

In the last three chapters we examined our world from a microscopic point of view. Now we can look at it from a macroscopic perspective.

Our world is full of life, both visible and invisible. All of these life forms are parts of the grand, integrated whole of nature, all interacting and sustaining the environment of our earth. In other words, all living organisms came from the same ancestor. The biological interactions are such that each and every one of the different plant and animal organisms of all sizes - from single-cell bacteria and algae to the great blue whale or the giant redwood - are helping each other in a beautiful system of interdependent harmony.

So many kinds of living organisms, millions of plants and animals, are living in different places in different ways. If we try to see some characteristics common to such a variety of living organisms, they might be:

1. Everything takes nutrition.
2. Everything grows.
3. Everything reproduces excessively.

The most important and interesting thing is the third point. Everything seems to be striving to increase. The speed at which this can happen is striking – a microbe can reproduce into the trillions within twenty-four hours. One single female salmon lays about fifty thousand eggs at one time. If all those babies survive, they can reproduce again in about two years. With enough food supplied, they would fill the entire ocean in ten years. One grain of corn grows and produces more than one to three thousand grains the first year; with enough nutrition, there will be more than one million the next year and two years later, a trillion. Here, too, within ten years the entire land surface of the earth would be covered with corn.

All other plants and animals are almost the same; their rate of growth would be the only difference. Generally speaking, the smaller living things increase more rapidly.

Competition between Living Organisms

The nutrition needed to sustain all living things comes from the earth; this includes water and air. Only green plants have the ability to synthesize these materials with the help of the sun's energy into organic forms of protein, fat, carbohydrates, and so on. These materials in turn become the nutrition for animals, which later return to the earth to provide nutrition for the plants themselves.

But competition does exist, not only between species but also between individuals of the same species. It comes into play both when organisms are seeking nutrition and when they are increasing and multiplying. Competition is found in its more severe form in the animal world, especially among humans during war. Plants and animals both compete for territory, and all animals share the same characteristic – to avoid being eaten. All animals require almost the same kind of nutrition – proteins, fats, and carbohydrates – but different species take nutrients from different kinds of foods, which helps reduce competition between species. Some animals eat only grasses, others only tree leaves. Still others eat a variety of grasses, roots, bark, and other parts of the plants, while some eat mainly animals; others eat both animals and plants.

Despite the diversity of feeding preferences, many species of animals still compete for the same food. Animals will fight to win in this fierce competition.

The herbivores don't need to fight or kill for their food because there is food in wide enough areas and the alert ones can get more if needed. If they attempt to dominate a larger territory, it is most often for purposes of sex and reproduction.

Carnivorous animals eat other animals, but there are not enough preys, so a more severe form of competition exists. Carnivorous animals must fight for their food. Leopards will catch antelopes or baboons; the lions will chase the leopards and rob them of their prey. Of all the carnivores, the lions and tigers seem to be the strongest and well deserving of the title "king of the beasts."

Elephants are herbivores and will not usually fight with other animals, but sometimes a carnivore will attack an elephant. Often this is not a good choice for the carnivore since lions are often defeated by elephants. Also, a pack of hyenas may attack and kill the kingly lion. So in this case, which is the stronger?

Food Pyramid

If we view the world as a place where fighting and competing are the rule, then what we are really illustrating is not the slogan "the strongest wins," but rather "the stronger eats the weaker."

The idea of the stronger eating the weaker, a predominant concept of the last several centuries, is a way of thinking that has supported such things as excessive meat-eating and conquest of other peoples. We feel we are the strongest, we can eat anything we want, we are the kings of the world. And truly, the last five hundred years has been the age of European dominance, spreading throughout the world.

About a hundred years ago the relationship between food and animals was pictured in the form of a food pyramid, as in the accompanying sketch.

Figure 8. Old Food Pyramid

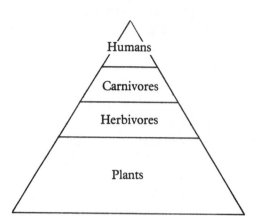

As research developed, questions were raised. With the discovery of microbes scientists came to realize these are also a kind of living thing and that they can kill human beings, animals, and plants. Thus they seem to be the strongest of all living things; in another way they are weak, as they are easily eaten by other tiny creatures.

The human species seems to be the weakest among animals in resisting the attack of microbes. People catch cold so easily, just from a cool wind or a slight dampness. Animals, on the other hand, can drink muddy water and eat food contaminated by flies. We cannot do this. Even a small cut on our skin or an insect bite can invite bacterial infection. The bacteria which cause syphilis and leprosy attack only the human body; they have no power to harm other animals. It seems the same with the AIDS virus.

As a result of microbial research, our food pyramid should be changed to look something like Figure 9. Nowadays the term food pyramid has been changed to food chain.

One Great Symbiosis
Seeing our world as a kind of battlefield is only one way to look

Figure 9. New Food Pyramid

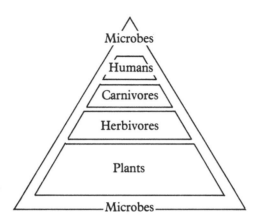

at it, and, with the kind of research that has developed, we have inclined to view our world in this way. But everything is also helping everything else, working and living together.

Animals eat plants, but they also help them to grow. Plants take in carbon dioxide and give off oxygen; animals take in oxygen and give back carbon dioxide for the plants. Plants produce honey in the flowers which serves as food for the insects. The bees, butterflies, and other insects eat the honey and at the same time assist in pollination, which is essential for some plant life. Birds eat fruit and berries and spread the seeds over a wide area. Animal excretions and dead bodies make good fertilizer for plants. This symbiotic relationship usually applies to two species of living things, but if we see all of nature in this way, the whole world is one great symbiosis. Everything is in harmony.

Herbivores eat plants, but at the same time they are controlling these plants so they do not take over. In the wild, some plants grow at such a rate that they finally cover a very dense area and appear to be flourishing. Then all of a sudden they die out, leaving the whole area barren except for the surrounding edges which stay alive. Botanists call this the phenomenon of the dead center. How this

happens is not really known – perhaps insufficient water or nutrition or too much heat. We just know that this sometimes happens.
But if animals eat the plants, this problem will not occur. (Of
course, wild animals never eat plants to the extent that none
remain.)

At one time the carnivores were considered undesirable because
they ate other animals and could possibly kill off all herbivores. But
now we know that carnivores are necessary links in natural systems.
Far from reducing the number of game animals, the carnivores
actually contribute to the stability of the food supply of game
animals. As a result of their niche in the system, individual animals
are better fed. This is a kind of contradiction, but our world itself
seems to consist of contradictions.

Sometimes rats multiply at an astounding rate. But then they
don't have enough food and go crazy, eating one another and moving out. Large numbers of rats form groups that move without
rhyme or reason or destination. They eat everything they meet on
their way. When they come to a river or beach, they continue on
into the water and die as if they had made a mass suicide pact.
However, if they were to be eaten by carnivorous animals before all
this happens, the problems created by the excessive rat population
could be avoided.

Food Shortages

At the beginning of this chapter I said that if anything reproduces in excess, competition between and within species increases.
Another result of overpopulation is the availability of more food for
other animals – an undesirable but inevitable consequence. Corn,
for example, is eaten by humans and animals; young salmon are
devoured by other fish. Things eat one another and this limits
overcrowding. In this way, our world remains harmonious and
balanced.

In early history human beings, too, were eaten by other animals;
as our ancestors grew stronger, this diminished. Then as populations

increased, food became limited and fighting arose in an attempt to resolve the problem. This started among families but progressed to clans, tribes, and even larger groupings, for people knew that a larger group is more powerful. Finally cities, countries, kingdoms, and empires arose, evolving into the great world communities.

Battles and Wars

People fought each other and took food and other necessities from one another. Leaders became kings and nobles, even taking their own people's food. Often more than half the crops cultivated by the peasants were taken away by the governors, a practice that eventually laid the groundwork for taxation.

It was through these taxes that the kings, nobles, and priests were enabled to live the good life and to train the more qualified young men to be their soldiers and professional fighters. So the people were afforded some protection by the king and his armies, but if the defense broke down, it was these same people who were forced to run for their lives. How many were killed in the fighting and its aftermath we have no way of knowing exactly – only that, after the histories were written down, the casualties suffered in this way were probably fewer than we think when compared with the total population.

About three hundred years ago in Europe the maximum number of soldiers that could be mobilized was about thirty thousand, for at that time the technology of transportation and machines was still relatively undeveloped. Beginning at the time of Napoleon, the scale of human war rose tremendously; about eight million died during World War I, and the total of war-related deaths related to World War II is estimated at more than twenty million, equal to about one percent of the world's population.

Famine and Plagues

More than wars, greater threats to populations have probably been famines, caused by drought, floods, or bad weather conditions which destroyed the crops. Starvation was not the only problem during these periods. Some died of food poisoning, trying to eat anything they could find, and others perished fighting over what little food remained. These are dark spots on the pages of human history. Some people even ate human flesh to survive. It is not a comfortable topic for discussion. We have no way of knowing the exact numbers of deaths directly related to the great famines, but we do know that they covered a wider area than wars, and killed more people.

The only reliable records come from the Great Famine which occurred in Europe (especially in Ireland) during the middle of the nineteenth century. The newly introduced potato crops were severely damaged by a plant disease known as the potato blight. About eight million people suffered and more than a million fled their native areas and migrated abroad, especially to the United States. An estimated 750,000 people, or 10 percent of the population of the affected area, died as a result of the famine.

Plagues took especially heavy tolls on the human population. In the middle of the sixth century history's worst, the Justinian Plague, began and remained in Europe and Asia Minor for some two hundred years, killing 100 million people. The Black Death broke out in Europe in the middle of the fourteenth century and about one-quarter of Europe's population, or twenty-five million people, perished within five years. During the same period the Plague spread into Africa and Asia. Some experts estimate that the world's population decreased by seventy million people, or more than 10 percent. Other plagues such as malaria, smallpox, cholera, typhus, and dysentery repeatedly affected the world population. Still, the human population has increased significantly.

Birth Control

In an attempt to avoid such disasters, people tried to limit the number of their children. Birth control is not new; one ancient record of contraception is contained in an Egyptian papyrus at least five thousand years old. Some Asians and American Indians used gromwell (*Radix Lithospermum* – "lithos" = stone, and "spermum" = seed or semen) for this purpose. We can assume from the botanical name that it was used by Europeans also. It is also likely that infanticide was widely practiced, although such practices were not usually recorded.

Table 12 provides an historical overview of the world's population development. From the time of Jesus Christ a span of 1,650 years was needed to double the human population. In another 160 years the original figure had quadrupled. It took 100 years more for the population to double again, bringing it to eight times the original number. It took another 60 years after the year 1900 for the population to double again. The principal reason for this slow growth of population was disease. Diseases have caused far greater damage to populations than either war or famine, and the greatest number of these have been infectious diseases.

Table 11. World Population Estimates

Year (A.D.)	Population
1	250,000,000
1000	340,000,000
1650	545,000,000
1800	907,000,000
1900	1,610,000,000
1950	2,509,000,000
1970	3,650,000,000

The Role of Disease

Surely diseases are terrible, but if wars recur today, it is possible that the whole world could be destroyed. At least disease is a kind of natural selection made by nature. Microbes attack everyone equally, although they can kill only the weak. But the point is, we can prevent disease. We can become stronger. It takes only a little bit of knowledge and a lot of practice; there is nothing difficult about it. Special tools or money are unnecessary. If anything, poorer people will find it easier.

The Romans

Let us look at some historical examples to see that the strongest and most powerful were also the most vulnerable to disease.

The ancient Romans were famous epicures and some of their menus have been recorded. It may surprise us to see what they ate. Nothing so unusual about beef and pork, but also fish, sea urchin, pigeon, deer, ostrich, flamingo, sweet cakes, and more – so many dishes at just one meal. If they had been healthy, their eating habits would be unimportant to us, but the average lifespan in ancient Rome, according to the Hungarian scholar J. Szilagyi, was 29.9 years. There were exceptions such as Cicero (63), Seneca (61), Galen (70), Plutarch (74), and Cato (85). This means that some had almost the same lifespan as modern people. The average life of Northern Africans at that time, 46.7, may be considered to be in the normal range; this was a general average in many countries prior to the last century.

If people die in their twenties, thirties, and forties, it is almost always from diseases, especially of the infectious type. These are the people most susceptible to microbes. The infant death rate among ancient peoples was also very high. Further, Roman law specified that a girl became an adult at the age of twelve. Many people married before they were fifteen and often became grand-parents at twenty-five. At thirty they were senior citizens. It is difficult to believe that such young parents could produce healthy babies. The great Roman Empire gradually lost power and finally ended in the sixth century.

The Peloponesian War

In 479 B.C. the Greek Athenians defeated the Persians and Athens became the most powerful city in the world and the trading center of Europe. Merchandise came from the East, from Egypt and other Mediterranean countries, and Athens became the richest city, with a strong military force and an especially powerful fleet of warships. Athens also became the cultural center of Europe, and many geniuses appeared in the fields of philosophy, literature, the arts, and many others. For the Greeks it was the second Golden Age, not seen since the time of Homer. The Athenians' overall contribution to human culture was tremendous.

But the Spartans were determined to take the leadership from the Athenians and formed the Peloponesian League which attacked Athens and her allies in 431 B.C. The Spartan army was strong but it had no financial support and no powerful navy, so it seemed unlikely they could win. But in 429 B.C. a terrible plague struck the Athenians' best troops and spread to the general citizenry. Thucydides wrote of it, "The disease was new, and disappeared as mysteriously as it came, afflicting only Athens and the most populous of the other towns."[1]

Strangely enough, this disease killed about a third of the Athenian army and a quarter of its citizens, but it did nothing to the Spartans or other peoples. What kind of infection was it, and can it be identified with any modern-day infection? From what we can infer from Thucydides, the disease clearly came from Egypt or Libya and was probably carried in fruit or meat. It could have been a combination of flu and salmonella or something similar. In Northern Europe we know that no salmonella appeared until the people ate imported foods in the sixteenth century. The Athenians ate mainly imported foods and probably became weak in their resistance to disease. They were also likely heavy meat-eaters.

The Spanish and the Aztecs

Even more mysterious was the collapse of the Aztec Empire in Mexico.

In 1519 Hernan Cortez, the commander of 500 Spanish soldiers, 100 sailors, and 16 horses, entered Aztec territory. At that time the population of the Aztec Empire was estimated to be 2.5 million. The army consisted of about 200,000 soldiers and reserve forces. Considering these figures it is difficult to imagine how Cortez could have conquered them, but it actually happened. Historians say that this was the most successful war ever fought in human history and that nothing can compare to it.

But no one explained how this victory was possible. Some say that the Spanish had developed weapons, but at that time the gun was still a very primitive instrument. The bullets only traveled three hundred feet and three to five minutes were needed to put in the next bullet and the gunpowder. And the Aztecs also had guns. Some claim that Cortez won because he resembled an Aztec god, but still this is not enough to explain his victory. The smallpox plague, carried to the New World by the Europeans, may have played an important role in the conquest. The main reason for this supposition is that the Aztec Indians had no immunity for this disease. But if this is true, why didn't they all die out? Historians estimate that only 10 to 15 percent died of the smallpox. If all the Indian population had died, we could say that they had no immunity, for this was virgin land for the smallpox. But many recovered and others were not affected. We can only say that these people had a weak immunity to the disease, meaning that their genes carried only a thin memory of the disease and/or their strength had deteriorated through eating bad food.

If the virgin land theory is correct, then southern Mexico was virgin land for the Spanish invaders also. Different weather conditions and many unfamiliar diseases existed such as yellow fever, malaria, yaws, and others. If the Aztec people had syphilis, why didn't the Spanish soldiers have the same problem? Many Aztec women had children by Spanish soldiers, yet the soldiers did not get syphilis. Before Cortez invaded Mexico, he contracted syphilis in Cuba, but within a few years he recovered mysteriously and completely, long before the cause or any treatments were known.

To me the most important factor was food. At that time the

Aztecs believed that their gods demanded human blood as a sacrifice. Each year there were five ceremonial days when more than fifteen thousand people were slaughtered. Michael Harner of the New School for Social Research recently proposed a theory based on the written documents of those times. He maintains that these sacrificed victims were eaten. But who ate them? Only the ruling elite and the warriors, as there was not enough for the entire population. Harner also cites accounts describing the fare of the poor who subsisted mainly on maize (corn) and beans, with an occasional turkey or dog.[2]

As the plague broke out it attacked the warriors first, leaving the Aztec forces depleted. Cortez allied himself with some Indian tribes but their forces of a couple of thousand men were but a small fraction of the Aztec forces. Eventually the Spanish conquest of southern Mexico was completed.

Spanish soldiers, like the Spartans, had been trained to do with a minimum of food. They had built up strong immune systems. No scurvy appeared on the Spanish ships, meaning that they must have eaten mainly grains and not much meat. Such a diet was Spanish tradition. Spain has a lot of barren land and people did not have enough feed for raising animals.

The Spanish Crown conferred on Cortez the title King of New Spain, but he rejected this honor and in 1529 returned to Spain with a great wealth of treasures. In the following year he returned to New Spain, but he found the country in a state of anarchy and many accusations were leveled against him. The fortunes of life are strange. Stripped of power, he returned to Spain and his life of misery began. It is difficult to believe, but he died a poor man in debt.

Powerful But Weak

The end of a hero's life is almost always miserable. Only a few of the lucky ones managed to become kings and pass on their crowns to their heirs. Also, royalty is not known for longevity; Alexander the Great, the first emperor of China, and many others died at a young age. The French Valois dynasty went through six kings in a hundred years, and the English Tudor family had five. The longest lasting dynasty in Russia, the Romanovs, provided Russian kings for about three hundred years; during this time there were eighteen kings, an average reign of seventeen years. All this suggests a pattern of short, unhealthy lives among the royalty. Likely, all the kings were heavy meat-eaters. Looking at their portraits painted by the great artists of the time, many of them look like a barrel with two arms. And, the king's position is almost always a dangerous one; how many were assassinated from the time of Julius Caesar to Louis XVI or Nicolas II?

Now, the kings of the animals – the carnivorous lions and the tigers – are nearing extinction. Two thousand years ago Chinese literature abounded in references to the tiger, but today there are no more tigers in the mountains of China; in India there are only a few. In Africa attempts are being made to protect the lion, but their propagation is still difficult.

Clearly, the principal cause for the decreasing animal population has been human invasion of their territories. No one would say that we ate the lions and the tigers, but we have cultivated their wild reserves for farms and livestock pastures. Many wild plants and herbivorous animals have lost their land also, in territories formerly shared with the carnivorous species. But even among animals the carnivores are disappearing faster than the herbivores. Likely, they too are weak in their resistance to disease; their lifespan is not so long compared to the herbivores, such as elephants and horses. Lions and tigers live for about fifteen to twenty years, while horses sometimes reach fifty and elephants one hundred years.

The marine world is also maintaining a kind of ecological harmony; dramatic decrease in the whale population through over-hunting is one problem, but other sea animals have decreased as well. Many sea animals are heavy meat-eaters. In a single day, for example, a blue whale will eat about two tons of krill (shrimp-like animals) or other small fish. Dolphins and sea lions are nearing extinction for the same reasons as land animals. Among populations of marine animals the heavy meat-eaters are the first to become extinct. (It is unlikely that people will stop fishing, as fish are such an important high-protein source, but if we try to eat more seaweed and less fish, the situation can be improved.)

At one time huge reptiles lived on the earth. For such enormous animals a very firm structure is required; if not, the body would be squashed down by its own sheer weight. Many of these reptiles were meat-eaters. It has been said that the cause of their extinction was a change in the earth's weather such that their food sources died out, but new research shows that the main problem for these animals was disease, especially diarrhea.

To maintain the harmony and balance of this world, nature has created nothing that is absolutely strong.

Consider the game of cards. People will not lose interest in a game if it is well designed. A deck of cards has four suits – diamonds, hearts, clubs, and spades – each of which has thirteen numbers, one to ten plus the jack, the queen, and the king. Generally the larger numbers are the stronger and the kings are the strongest of all. But if the king simply beat everything in the deck, the game would be uninteresting and quickly finished. So the game is designed such that the lowest number one, the ace, can defeat the king. The spade is the symbol of peasants and considered the lowest class, but the ace of spades often becomes the most powerful card.

Victorious Microbes

Nature has made our world somewhat the same. Now, the microbial world is showing its strength. Scientists are warning that artificial nitrogen fixation, a technology which has greatly increased our food production through factory-made ammonia, nitrates, and nitrites, has limited the natural nitrogen in the air. Microbes are so sensitive that, with even a minimal amount of material change in the world, they react immediately and start to adjust to maintain balance. Now, nitrifying bacteria are decreasing and denitrifying bacteria are increasing. Even if we produce more fertilizer, nitrifying bacteria will not increase. Again the microbes seem to be victorious over humans.

What we have learned is that eating animal food makes the body strong for fighting but weak for the attacks of microbes. Strong empires collapse more from the inside than from invading enemies, mainly due to physical deterioration from eating rich food. By the same token the richest people are often the most unhealthy.

Chapter 14

Plant and Animal Foods

You Are What You Eat

We hear it said, "You are what you eat." Is this statement true or not? It is ridiculous to think that if someone eats pork and beans he will become like a pig or a bean. Our body breaks down all the food we take in and reduces it to the molecular stage, and only these materials are used for making blood, cells, and everything else. Our muscles are not made of pork. We can see, however, that vegetarians tend to look a little different than meat-eaters, especially over many years. Generally speaking, vegetarians are thinner and their skin color is lighter; meat-eaters tend to have bigger and heavier bodies, often with a dark or red color.

If we eat oranges or orange juice, carrots, or pumpkins every day for one or two months, an orange color will show on the palms of our hands. If we eat beets, a purple color will appear in the urine. If we eat an excessive amount of oil over a long period of time, a yellow color can be found just beneath the skin; it cannot be seen on the surface, but if you press your palms and they appear yellow, it means excess oils (fat) were taken in.

Surely, foods influence us a great deal, not only physically but also mentally and emotionally. Research in this area has not been fully developed, but here I would like to look at the influence of

foods, especially plant and animal foods, and how each relates to us.
Our diet consists almost entirely of plants and animals and of foods
derived from both groups. These are the largest classifications
among the food groups.

Plants Grow Upward

It is characteristic of plants to grow upward toward the sky as
they stretch out their branches and stems. Flowers, leaves, and
fruits grow on the top part or near the end of branches, so they, too,
show a tendency to go upward. Nutrition, energy, and growth –
everything seems related to an upward direction. If plants compete
with each other, they tend to become taller and taller.

Plants manufacture carbohydrates. Monosaccharides, the simplest form of carbohydrates, are found only in the flower and the
fruit. Monosaccharides are the main component of honey and they
also account for the sweet taste of fruit. Plants concentrate monosaccharides to disaccharides and send these throughout the entire
body of the plant, making cellulose and starch, and forming a solid
and sturdy character. Cellulose is a complex carbohydrate, as is
starch, another product manufactured by the plant. This is stored
mainly inside the fruits and seeds; often it is carried below the
surface and stored in the roots or tubers of the plant.

Flowers, fruits, and leaves fall to the ground after they die.
Seeds are different; they are still living after they fall and can
produce new plants. Therefore, seeds and roots are different in
character from other parts of the plant. Instead of going upward,
they tend to go downward, or seek the ground, which seems closer
to the behavior of animals.

All animals are warm-bodied, except for the primitive ones.
Maintaining optimal body temperature means that the body cannot
be stretched as plants can be stretched. To protect against heat loss,
an animal's body grows as a mass: the blood circulates throughout
the entire body and the skin, muscles, bones, and inner organs
grow almost simultaneously. The human body grows more

Figure 10. Human Body Growth

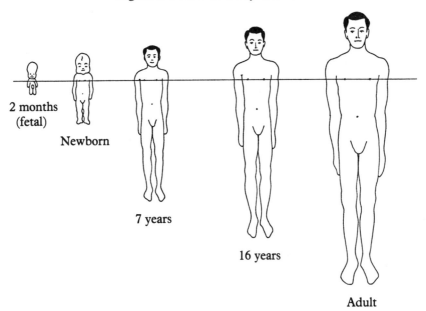

2 months
(fetal)

Newborn

7 years

16 years

Adult

downward than upward, as illustrated. The body is heavy by nature and needs to lie down; it takes effort for animals to keep their bodies upright for their activities.

Opposite Energy

Briefly put, plant energy goes up and animal energy goes down, and they have opposite characteristics. More of the vegetal nutrition goes to the upper parts of our body to feed the body cells found there; at the same time, taking an excess of this same plant nutrition may damage that part of the body. The nutrients in animal food tend to become good nutrition for the lower parts of our body, but here too an excess will result in damage to those areas. I cannot say this very strictly, as the blood circulates in the whole body and feeds all the body cells, which need a combination of nutrients. But in the blood, heavier and lighter materials do exist and they have separate tendencies. For example, alcohol, vinegar,

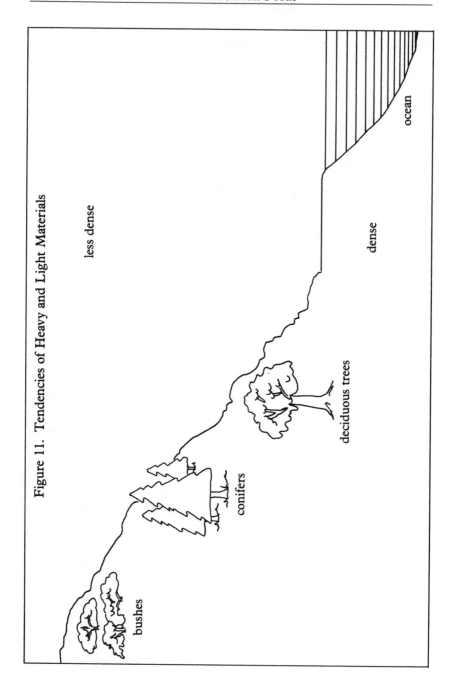

Figure 11. Tendencies of Heavy and Light Materials

and hot spices, all derived from plants, are substances that go to the upper part of our body, often causing the head to sweat or affecting brain function. Animal foods, on the other hand, will affect the lower body, stimulating sexual desire, for example.

In our modern scientific world this concept may seem strange or unique, but it provides definite answers to many enigmas and mysteries in medical research. In the accompanying illustration (Figure 11) we can see that this is just common sense: heavy materials go down and stay, light materials rise and disperse. The two tendencies are often mixed together so that slight differentiations occur at any particular time. However, over time it makes a big difference if one tendency is continually over-used. But we have to understand a little more about the body.

In Figure 12 we have pictures of a complete body, a head, a trunk, a leg, and the pupil of the right eye. In the practice of iridology the pupil reveals almost all parts of the body. The relationship of upper to lower exists throughout the entire body; upper parts of one section relate to upper parts of another section, such as brain, forehead, and lungs with the upper part of the legs. In the face, the mouth area relates to the lower abdomen. Dividing the body into even smaller units, the same relationships exist, even at the level of individual cells. But to avoid confusion, it is necessary to understand only that every upper part is related to every other upper part, and every lower part is connected with every other lower part at every level throughout the body.

The Best Nutrient Is the Most Harmful

Viewed in one way, we could assume that the best nutrition for the brain would be honey, which is from the very top of the plants just as the brain is located at the top of the body. But I have found that many brain tumor and cancer patients have been great lovers of honey. Alcohol also damages the brain, but it evaporates quickly; except in cases of continuous abuse, its damage may even be less than that of honey or other concentrated sweeteners. After honey,

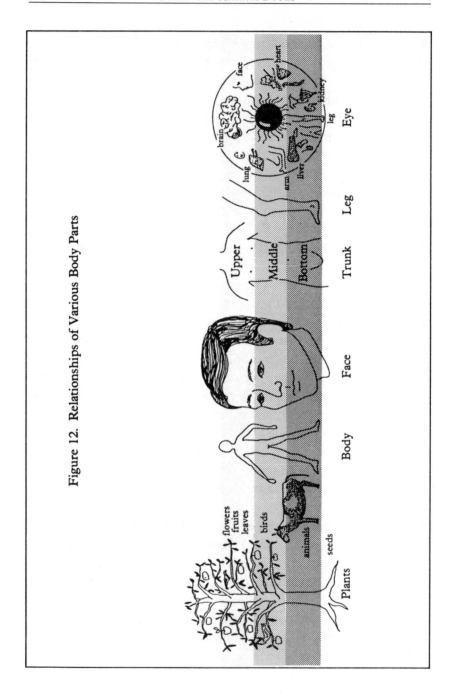

Figure 12. Relationships of Various Body Parts

sugar seems to have the most powerful effect on the brain. This may seem strange at first, since sugar comes from the whole sugar cane (or beets) and is not found only at the top of the plant, but the concentrated sugar cane juice rises to the top in the refining process, thereby sharing the same upward characteristic. After sugar, maple syrup, corn syrup, and other concentrated sweeteners also have the same characteristics as honey and sugar but in a slightly weaker form. All of them, however, strongly affect the brain and the nervous and respiratory systems, all of which are located mainly in the upper part of the body.

Brain Damage

One of the most difficult diseases of human history has been rabies. The virus attacks the brain and nervous system almost exclusively; rarely is there any infection in the area bitten by a rabid dog. The virus passes slowly through the body and tends to rise, causing definite damage to the brain and nervous system. The question is, why did rabies suddenly become so prevalent in the seventeenth and eighteenth centuries? The ancient Greeks had written about the disease many centuries before, but no records were found in northern Europe during this later time period. Due to longer flowering seasons, countries in southern Europe produced more honey; for those in the north, honey was an expensive luxury. After the time of Alexander the Great, sugar was imported from Asia into Greece. By the seventeenth century sugar had become popular in Europe and incidences of rabies suddenly increased. Even if the disease was caused by the virus, the most significant co-factor was the consumption of honey and sugar. The rabies virus seems to be chasing sugar-rich nutrition. Also, many other kinds of encephalitis are related to the intake of the sweetest foods.

In the past some bacteria were known as a causative agent of brain disease, but the incidence was not high except for syphilis. In recent years, viral research has developed and many viruses have been identified as the cause. The favorite host cells for the virus seem to be the brain and nerve cells. These neurotropic viruses have a tendency to seek the upper body.

The causal relationship between honey and sugar and diseases of the brain and nervous system is fairly easy to understand, but other diseases are more complicated. Many kinds of bacteria and viruses cause disease, and so many different foods can be co-factors. Therefore, again I will offer a simple classification according to food groups.

Ascending and Descending Energy

In the category of animal foods, the meat of mammals – what we know as red meat – produces the strongest effects. Then come eggs, chicken, and the meat of other fowl, followed by white meat fish, shrimp, shellfish and other primitive sea animals, whose effects are somewhat weaker. The weakest foods in this category are milk and other dairy products, whose characteristics are close to those of plant foods.

How these foods affect us can be shown by one common example. Teenagers often have acne and pimples, which may appear only on the forehead, only in the middle of the face, only around the lower part of the mouth, or sometimes over the whole face. These occur at the time of hormonal change, but certain dietary factors can be correlated to these locations. Pimples appearing at the lower part of the face relate to the consumption of red meat; those at the middle of the face to chicken and eggs; those at the lower part of the forehead to primitive sea animals; and those at the very top of the forehead to dairy products.

Among plant foods, after honey and sugar, fruits have the most ascending energy, then vegetables, next beans, then large nuts and seeds. Small seeds and grains have the least. Grains have a more neutral character but are not as effective as vegetables in balancing the descending energy and helping to neutralize the waste products of animal foods. Sugar also has no cleansing effect in this way. Each food group provides conditions favorable for certain bacterial infection, but by combining categories these effects are neutralized to a certain degree. Most everyone eats an omnivorous combination of plant and animal foods; pure vegetarians or carnivores are rare.

Two Forms of Disease

Typical tuberculosis is a lung disease affecting the upper part of the body. The brain, the lungs, and the nervous system are all weakened by excessive eating of plant foods, sugar especially. Bacteria always attack and damage the weakest parts of the body, in this case the lungs and nervous system. In the seesaw game of meat and sugar the bacteria will go to other parts of the body – such as the kidneys or the skin – and create different forms of disease in these areas.

As we saw in an earlier chapter, common leprosy is related to an excess consumption of animal food. Tuberculoid leprosy, on the other hand, is the sign of an excessive intake of plant food. But the question remains, why in sixteenth century Europe did leprosy begin to decrease at the same time tuberculosis increased? One theory speculates that the bacteria which cause leprosy and tuberculosis are very similar (belonging to the same family) and compete with each other; if one type (tuberculosis) enters the body, the body gains immunity to the other (leprosy). Also, the tuberculosis bacteria can be spread from host to host through the air as the patient sneezes or coughs, while the leprosy bacteria can be transmitted only by direct bodily contact; this gave tuberculosis a distinct advantage. After the bubonic plague of the fourteenth century, the practice of one person per bedroom became common. People had less opportunity to touch each other's bodies.

Recent medical research suggests that the amount of vitamin C from plant foods in the diet may also have been of some importance in the decline of leprosy, for vegetables contain vitamin C which helps to neutralize toxicity of meat. But vegetable consumption does not increase tuberculosis significantly. I think the most important factor in the development of tuberculosis was increased sugar consumption. Tuberculosis began to spread in the sixteenth century when the Portuguese and the Spanish were navigating the high seas and trading commodities with the East. This coincided with Fracastoro's theory of germs which had a great influence in southern Europe. In 1546 Paracelsus published his clinical study of tuberculosis indicating an increasing incidence of this disease. Then in the middle of the seventeenth century there was a sudden outbreak of tuberculosis in England. In 1662 the English had imported some 16 million pounds of sugar and other European countries followed soon after. European people aquirred so many acute diseases as a result of eating imported foods that before the patients were identified, they had succumbed to another disease. In this way the leprosy bacteria almost disappeared without spreading (see Table 13).

As I wrote earlier, the Black Death or pestis also came in two forms. *Tuberculoid pestis* was caused by excessive consumption of plant food; in the fourteenth century the populations of Eastern countries contracted this form of pestis as a result of eating sugar and honey. The second form of pestis – the bubonic plague (the type that almost all European victims had) – was caused by excessive meat consumption. There was a third form of pestis – septecemic pestis – fundamentally not much different from the second type; extremely large amounts of both animal and plant foods were eaten, so that over a period of time high levels of toxic materials accumulated in the blood. When bacteria invaded such a body, they were able to increase with great rapidity and destroy the body cells.

Interestingly, plant food produces stronger effects on the left side of the body than on the right. For example, if excessive meat consumption is the cause of paralysis, the paralysis will usually appear suddenly in the form of a stroke which affects the right side over the left. At the age of 46 Louis Pasteur was paralyzed. Using the theory of Oriental diagnosis I am assuming this was mainly in his left hand and arm. He was a genius, but he probably never

Table 12. First Records of Diseases in Europe
(numbers indicate century)

Disease	Causative Agent	Known to have existed B.C.	Italy Spain	Other European Countries	Peak
malaria	protozoa	yes	A.D. 16	A.D. 16	A.D. 19
pneumonia	various	yes	–	17	20
dysentery	protozoa bacteria	yes	6	6	19
tuberculosis	bacteria	yes	–	16	19
leprosy	bacteria	yes	6	6	14
syphilis	bacteria	no	15	16	19
diptheria	bacteria	yes	15	16	19
typhoid fever	bacteria	yes	–	17	19
cholera	bacteria	no	16	16	19
scarlet fever	bacteria	no	14	16	19
smallpox	virus	yes	16	16	17
measles	virus	yes	14	14	19
German measles	virus	no	–	17	19
polio	virus	yes	–	18	20
rabies	virus	yes	13	16	19
yellow fever	virus	no	–	17	19-20
English sweats	unknown	no	–	16	16
cancer	unknown	yes	–	6	20
diabetes	unknown	yes	–	16	20
gout	unknown	yes	15	16	20
osteoporosis	unknown	no	–	17	20
arthritis	unknown	yes	–	3	20
rheumatic fever	unknown	yes	16	17	20

considered his high sugar consumption to be a cause of his disease. Pasteur carried out much of his great research with a paralyzed body. This was an amazing achievement for which a very strong will power must have been needed. As another example, the newly developed diagnostic technique of thermography shows that the right side of a normal body emits more heat than the left side.

Diseases of Heavy Meat-Eaters

Diseases typically associated with excessive meat-eating are gout, gangrene, and classic Kaposi's sarcoma. When Moriz Kaposi described this rare form of tumor, the patients were all male and the disease first appeared in the foot. Gout and gangrene, too, almost always begin in the foot and more often appear on the right side of the body. This is just the opposite of the symptoms that arise from excessive consumption of plant food.

Gout was a common affliction in Roman times. According to the *Hippocratic Aphorisms,* sex was a co-factor in the development of gout and castration was even proposed as a remedy. Royal families and the highest classes of society were especially prone to this "royal disease." Later, it became common everywhere in Europe when meat consumption had increased. Today in the United States about two million people are afflicted with gout. Medical research has discovered that gout is caused by excessive uric acid in the blood from improperly metabolized protein purine. A more difficult problem than the disease itself may be that people still wish to consume excess animal protein.

A diabetic ulcer is a more complicated form of trouble. The main cause is excess sugar, but also a large amount of meat. As a result, the ulcer often starts from the underside of the big toe (lower body).

All these kinds of diseases are suppurative (purulent) forms or similar. On the other hand, sugar or honey cause infections that are almost always associated with the respiratory organs like the common cold or flu. Depending on how much sugar is consumed, there can be afflictions of the brain and nervous system.

Other opposed characteristics between plant and animal foods are shown in Table 14.

Animals Are Warm

As you see in Table 14, plants are cool and animals are warm. Mammals and birds have especially warm bodies. Certain tempera-

Table 14. Characteristics of Plants and Animals

Characteristic	Plants	Animals
temperature	cold	warm
taste	sweet, sour, hot	salty
smell	fragrant	stinks
color	green	red
size	tall	long and wide
body fluid	water	blood
activity	stationary	movement
sound	quiet	noisy
weight	light	heavy
nervous system	unknown	strong
minerals	potassium	sodium
	calcium	phosphorous
	magnesium	sulfur
lifespan	long life	short life

tures are required for physical activity; our muscles cannot move quickly if conditions are too cold. When we sleep, our body temperature is slightly lower for the cells are less active and we need less energy. Certain mammals can lower their body temperature by more than twenty degrees when they hibernate in the winter time, but if something frightens them, their temperature suddenly rises again and they can run. Even the body temperature of ocean fish is not the same as the water they swim in, each species having a little different temperature, in the area of 75°F.

We receive plenty of energy from the sun every day, but we have no way to store it; water can hold a little of the heat energy from the sun, but this heat is quickly dissipated. Neither can other inorganic materials hold on to this energy for very long. But plants can convert the sun's energy into their own bodies and conserve it for a long time. In this form the sun's energy is stable and can be transported from one place to another. Only green plants have the ability to synthesize energy in organic form.

If we say that plants are a concentrated form of the sun's energy, then herbivorous animals are an even more concentrated form of it. It is said that more than eight times the energy of plants is concentrated in an animal's body by weight. Our body heat also originates from the sun through the eating of plants.

Plants Are Cooler

With dried plants, such as wood, we can make fire; the plant's heat energy is released in this way, but the source of the energy was originally the sun. Even coal, petroleum, and natural gases are plants or animals as found in changed forms; the energy of these fuels also originated from the sun.

Plants usually maintain a temperature that is colder than the air. Even under the summer sun their leaves do not become hot in comparison with other materials. Water is constantly evaporating from the leaves and keeping them cool. At night the leaves collect moisture from the air, forming water droplets and helping the roots to take in water. The plant's body is a kind of radiator.

Animal bodies are naturally warm. We are consumers of the sun's energy. Warmer-bodied animals consume more food and are more active. Reptiles have varying body temperatures, but usually they are much cooler than mammals, and they move more slowly. Humans consume ten times more food than many kinds of reptiles.

Animal Foods Warm the Body

If we eat meat we can feel the warmth in our hands, feet, and head. For this reason, meat-eaters can easily get high fevers. Poultry especially is known to produce warmth; many people prefer to eat chicken, turkey, goose, and other fowl in winter. The meat of birds can cause higher fevers than the meat of mammals. The temperature of fish is lower and so is less likely to cause a high fever. Plant food will never produce a high fever. If pure vegetarians do get a fever, it will be low, usually about 100°F to 102°F at most. Their bodies can defeat microbes without high temperature; they don't need it. However, if they contract a brain disease from eating too much sugar or honey and no warming animal foods, and if the microbes attack the brain only, then this is dangerous for pure vegetarians as the brain cells don't produce heat. For those who eat meat, the fever needed to defeat the microbes is produced by the high octane animal foods.

The Calorie Theory

This relationship of food to heat poses some questions in regard to the calorie theory. Calories are measured by burning food as a fuel, as if you were burning firewood, gasoline, or coal in order to measure the amount of heat produced. The calorie is almost solely the product of carbon as it combines with oxygen to give off heat. But an animal's body is not so simple; we generate heat in a different way than wood stoves do.

The caloric energy of animal foods is commonly considered to be derived from oils or fats; when we eat these foods the body usually becomes warmer and more active. Nuts also contain large amounts of oil, yet they do not tend to heat the body so much. So the resolution of the calorie question must be found not only in the fat, but the protein as well. Also, animal proteins seem to make the body warmer whereas plants (such as soybeans) have no significant effect.

Cattle producers feed their stock soybeans; statistically it takes about sixteen pounds of soybeans to produce one pound of beef. Is much energy and protein lost or concentrated? Perhaps both. At least it is sure that the animal body is a more concentrated form of energy than that of plants.

There are quick-burning fuels like straw and slow-burning fuels such as coal, and also there are high-temperature-producing fuels like coal and gasoline as well as low-temperature-producing fuels like wood. Our foods are similar. Plant foods are slow-burning in the body while meat (especially poultry) which requires and stores high octane fuels makes the body feel warm, under normal conditions.

Differing Body Temperatures

Meat-eaters, having warmer body temperatures as a result of the energy in animal foods, tend to be more active, are sometimes noisy, often engage in physical work, and often change locations. If you eat a lot of meat and are not active, toxins can quickly build up and invite disease. Athletes or body builders have tended to be meat-eaters, although many are finding that complex carbohydrates provide better stamina and a cooler head.

Vegetarians, on the other hand, have slightly lower body temperatures and will tend to be more passive and quiet, staying in one place for longer periods of time. This kind of diet is favored by those who do more mental work such as thinking, meditating, writing, etc. Some notable examples are Pythagoras, Plato, Jean-Jacques Rousseau, Albert Einstein, Leo Tolstoy, and many writers, philosophers, and religious people throughout history.

Often a vegetarian diet was emphasized for spiritual development. The ancient Egyptians showed in their art that the upper part of the human body differed from that of the animals, while the lower part remained the same; it has been universally recognized that the human being's special abilities lie in the upper part of the body. Sylvester Graham and others taught that if we eat meat our body becomes sexually overactive and we risk losing our special human abilities. Others, especially in religion, have referred to the sex drive as the "beastly desire." This is overstated, but something to consider. The special human abilities are creativity, thinking, loving, social relationships, self-denial, and more, but almost everything is connected to mental activity.

Food and Behavior

Emotions, too, are greatly influenced by diet. Meat-eaters are generally more emotional, showing extremes of anger, sadness, laughter, crying, and shouting. Sylvester Graham said that too much animal food makes man easily angered and aggressive. Fear and sadness seem to appear without any provocation. People express these kinds of emotions through "fight or flight." Anger leads to fighting and fear to fleeing. Both of these emotions are controlled mainly by the adrenal glands. On the other hand, worry and sadness can result from an excess of plant foods. These emotions stay in the brain for a long time, often leading to more fatigue and stress. A typical reaction of this condition is weeping, quite different from crying and shouting.

How are food and human behavior related? This kind of scientific research started only ten years ago. Studies on how caffeine affects brain activity and how tryptophan, choline, and other elements activate brain cells have been conducted. Surely food has a relationship with human behavior.

Here I would like to correct a misconception about the relationship between food and activity. Most people believe that sugar makes children hyperactive, but this conclusion is based on a short-term observation. If children are fed with enough protein and then sugar is added, they will become hyperactive. However, if protein is low and they are given a lot of sugar, children become quiet, low in energy, pale, always tired, and may often catch cold. A slightly anemic condition can be the first stage of a serious illness such as tuberculosis. Even small amounts of sugar over a long period can cause trouble (for vegetarians or anyone), so be careful of slow-progressing problems. When the effects are recognized, often it is too late for a good recovery. One thing to remember is that sugar has no power to neutralize the acids that result from eating meat. Also, sugar today is highly refined and processed and thus more dangerous. If we can control AIDS and other infections by giving up sugar, it might be a fair exchange.

It is characteristic of plants and plant-eaters that they change slowly. Meat-eaters, on the contrary, go through physical, mental, and emotional changes very quickly. It is the same with disease. The symptoms and conditions of meat-eaters will change quickly, sometimes for the worse, sometimes for the better, while the vegetarian's condition changes more slowly. Vegetarians may not die so suddenly, but once a disease takes hold in their body, it is also harder to cure in a short period of time.

Food Over Psychology

Studies in psycho-neuro-immunology have demonstrated that the brain and the immune system make up a closed circuit. The brain's chemicals regulate immune defenses. The immune system also sends chemical messages about bacteria and viruses to the brain. The brain controls the whole body – the heartbeat, body temperature, and so on – so that our psychological condition can have a powerful effect in fighting a disease. This is the new research of mind over malady. This is very interesting, but we must go one more step forward: the quality of the blood has a strong influence on the brain, and the quality of blood is determined mainly by our food. This actual fact should not be overlooked in research studies. My opinion is that food precedes and leads us to certain psychological conditions. Even psychological problems can be controlled by food to a certain degree and sometimes completely.

It is said that some disease is caused by great stress, but we need not have such stress; the brain itself has a built-in protective mechanism. If we try to overuse the brain, it will automatically begin to sabotage us by cloudy thinking, difficulty in concentration, loss of memory, and drowsiness. Yawning, deep breathing, or nodding are forced on us by the brain if we are overworked. If we take sugar, coffee, tea, or some kind of drug in order to continue, it will enable us to go far beyond our usual limits, but headaches and other maladies will result.

The Sugar-Iron Connection

Has sugar, then, made no contribution whatever to human life? It has, indeed, probably a big one. In the last several centuries many geniuses have appeared. These are the sugar geniuses – Pasteur, Shelley, Mozart, Beethoven, Tchaikovsky, Van Gogh, and many more. However, many of our geniuses have also been weak physically and some mentally. The high sugar of fruits can also bring these effects. If we go back to even earlier times, the factors that caused the simultaneous appearance of so many geniuses in ancient Greece during the Pericules Age may have had some relationship with honey, which the Greeks imported from Africa and the East and used widely.

But the Athenians also suffered a huge loss during the Peloponesian War, mainly because of the attack of an epidemic. Thucydides wrote that the disease came from Egypt or Libya. I think imported food caused this disease and the failure of the Athenians.

Almost at the same time, many geniuses surfaced in China and India. The Chinese knew about honey very early but did not produce much; sugar was unknown. The Indians had sugar, so this was not a new development. Another factor helped to create many geniuses like Confucius and Gautama Buddha: I think the iron pot for cooking was an important contribution to the making of genius.

Travel from ancient Greece to India and China was limited, but the introduction of iron pots for cooking coincided in these three areas. Iron is the essential element for making hemoglobin which carries oxygen from the lungs to the body cells. The brain uses a lot of oxygen for its activity. Scientific researchers now say that using iron pots for cooking can prevent anemia. And iron is not dangerous like sugar and honey. We should begin to use iron pots once again.

Salt Balances Plant Foods

Some interesting new research says that plants have a kind of nervous system, but the function is much different than in an animal's body. Plants do not have enough sodium for a nerve impulse. If we compare the composition of plants and animals, we find that many elements are the same in both, but there is an extreme shortage of sodium and chlorine in plants. If we eat plant food only, we too will be short on these two elements. Salt contains both sodium and chlorine, so it is the perfect supplementary food for vegetarians. A shortage of sodium or an excess of potassium will create a malfunction of the nervous system.

Salt is neither animal food nor plant food, but a mineral. This unique ingredient is a counterbalance to plant food, creating harmony in the body. Since salt is heavy, it tends to encourage a downward direction as animal foods do, but salt, unlike animal foods, does not create acidity in the body.

Mysterious Disease

Although it is not a comfortable subject to discuss, being a food researcher it is my obligation to report to you the most dangerous food.

A small tribe called the Fore are living in the eastern highlands of New Guinea. Around the middle of this century a terrible brain disease called kuru became an epidemic among these people; within about one year of the onset of the disease, 100 percent of the patients died.

Many medical people have an interest in such unknown diseases, so some of them heard this news and went there to study kuru. If this had been a kind of infection, then some of the neighboring peoples might have shared the same trouble, but this was not found to be the case. Food poisoning, allergy, malnutrition, and hereditary factors were examined but the disease did not fit into any category. After many attempts in animal testing, some researchers finally inoculated a chimpanzee brain with the brain cells of a kuru patient and produced a very similar disease. Inoculation from this diseased brain to another healthy chimpanzee brain was successful and the transmissibility of the disease was established.

The Fore were still practicing a very unusual tradition in this twentieth century: they ate the human bodies of deceased members of the tribe. During the funeral all the relatives came together, made a fire, and burnt the body. When it was half burnt, they took the body out of the fire and ate it. At the peak of the epidemic about 6 percent of all deaths among the Fore were caused by kuru.

And the disease was more prevalant among women and children than among men.

The government received the doctor's report and prohibited the cannibalism immediately. Within several years the incidence of the disease decreased dramatically, but some questions still remain. Why were women and children more susceptible to the trouble? I am assuming that the main job of handling the dead body belonged to the men. Likely, the men ate the steak first and the women and children ate the leftovers, mainly the inside organs and the brain. Those who ate the diseased brain had the most trouble.

But why did this disease became such an horrible epidemic in the middle of this century even though this tribe and their ancestors had practiced this tradition for a long time, perhaps thousands of years? This is easy to understand because in this century they began to eat sugar and other imported foods. If scientists could understand the relationship between sugar and brain disease, many difficult problems could be resolved.

About thirty years have passed since the peak of this disease and today kuru is identified only in rare cases and then exclusively among the elderly. Doctors suggest that these patients had been exposed to the virus some twenty or thirty years before. Since both viruses are lentiviruses, AIDS encephalopathy is most similar to kuru disease. Many AIDS researchers admit that it is possible to have a long incubation time with AIDS, as with kuru.

Another mysterious brain disease, Creitzfeld-Jakob disease, was discovered in the early 1920s and was also fatal. This is now understood as being caused by the same category of virus. Although the transmission route has not yet been proven, some reports say that it comes from people in northern Africa and the Mediterranean countries who eat sheep (lamb), especially if they eat the brain.

Scrapie and AIDS

Scrapie is a kind of sheep disease that affects the brain, the nervous system, and some of the respiratory system of humans. It has been known in Europe for almost three hundred years, but the cause and treatment are unknown. What is known is that it is contagious and 100 percent lethal. The earliest symptom of this disease occurs when the infected sheep scrape their itchy skin against any convenient object. The only way to control the spread of this disease is to kill all suspicious sheep and bury them. Now, scrapie is spreading from sheep to goats, cows, and other animals.

From the similarities of kuru, Creitzfeld-Jakob disease, and scrapie, Dr. John Seale, a famous British venerologist, proposed a new theory about the origin and the transmission route of AIDS. He suggests that the scrapie virus has invaded the human body and is the cause of AIDS, and thus AIDS has no relationship with sexual activity. It is too early to say if this is correct or not, but few people accept this theory. However, we can draw the conclusion that if we eat meat, the chance of getting an infectious disease is much higher.

According to Dr. Thomas G. Hull humans share 65 types of diseases with dogs; 50 with cows; 46 with sheep or goats; 42 with pigs; 35 with horses; 32 with rats and mice; and 26 with poultry. You can see that the closer to humans the animals are, the more diseases are shared. We share the same environment and similar foods.

The Most Dangerous Food

Why did humans give up the practice of eating human flesh very early, maybe tens of thousands of years ago? I can find no law which prohibits cannibalism except for the one in New Guinea. Many religious teachings say not to eat animal meat, but they never say not to eat human flesh. This is beyond laws or morals, and should be a needless discussion for anyone. But I think our ancestors had a similar experience as the Fore people and human flesh was not eaten based on fear of disease and the tradition that followed. Next to human flesh, animal meat is the most dangerous food.

The next question is: if the sheep did not eat sugar or meat, how did they contract such an awful disease as scrapie? I think it was caused by chemicals in man-made paper, which they sometimes ate without knowing any better. This unusual food caused a viral mutation, and this became the scrapie virus; it was an accident.

Two hundred years later humans began adding chemicals to their own food intentionally. Colors, preservatives, flavors, lubricants, stabilizers, thickeners, fumigants, sweeteners, and many more are now widely used. Moreover, many chemicalized medical drugs are being consumed. Due to the last one hundred years of experimentation, human society is now rampant with brain diseases and mental troubles.

If you agree with my opinion, then don't eat any risky foods such as sugar, animal meat, or chemicalized foods, starting today.

Chapter 15

Body Balance
and Central Control

We Eat Electricity

You may think I am crazy for saying that we eat electricity, but this is not a new discovery. Already much scientific research has been done. I have only changed the expression. If I use the term electrolytes, then the meaning is more clear. Our body is functioning by electricity, especially in the brain and nervous system. Since electrolytes are in our food and in our bodies, forming electric current, this means we are eating electricity.

Any material can be divided into molecules, which are composed of groups of atoms. An atom is composed of protons, neutrons, and electrons. Electrically, protons have a positive charge and are housed in the neucleus with the neutrons. The surrounding electrons have a negative charge and as a whole the atom is ordinarily neutral.

Water is composed of two hydrogen atoms and one oxygen atom. We can think of pure water as just plain water, but actually it is more complicated. The water molecules break up and form hydrogen ions (H^+) and hydroxyl ions (OH^-). Water is always the mixture of these ions and molecules that are not ionized. There are some thirty trillion hydrogen ions and the same number of hydroxyl ions in a milliliter of water in addition to sixty billion times that number of molecules that are not ionized. The ions combine again and other molecules form new ions and are always changing back and forth. But still the water is electrically neutral and water by itself does not conduct electrical current.

Common table salt is also electrically neutral, but when dissolved in the water, sodium ions (Na^+) and chlorine ions (Cl^-) separate and can conduct electrical current. When a substance is dissolved in water and breaks down into ions, these are called electrolytes. Among the most important electrolytes in our bodies are hydrogen (H^+), sodium (Na^+), potassium (K^+), magnesium (Mg^+), calcium (Ca^+), chlorine (Cl^-), sulfur (S^-), phosphorus (P^-), oxygen (O^-), iodine (I^-), the hydroxyl ion (OH^-), bicarbonate (HCO_3^-), and carbonate (CO_3^-).

Electricity has two poles, positive and negative. Their character is opposite and they attract each other in working together and making balance. The biological current is very weak, about 40 to 120 millivolts, but is essential energy for life. The electrolytes are experienced as the tastes of acid and alkaline. After food is absorbed by the body, we cannot feel the electrolytes, but these are the main forces involved in body balancing.

The Body's Balance

In this world, everything is harmonious and balanced and so the word "balance" is often used. In our body there is water, nitrogen, and hormone balance; when we inhale and exhale, air creates balance; and our nutrition should be balanced with our activity in terms of input and output. If we lose the balance between the right and left sides of the body, we fall. This is the original meaning of balance. The children's seesaw game is a good example. To keep balance, each side alternates in opposite directions; with only one child, the game cannot be played. If both children come toward the center of the board and hug each other, the board can become level and perfectly balanced, but actually this seldom happens. So when we say "balance," there are always two underlying forces, opposite or antagonistic directions, that are working together to adjust extreme imbalance.

It is easy to understand that our body is maintaining good health and proper functioning by perfect balance. But before we go on to the subject of central control, it is necessary to understand acid and alkaline balance.

Acid and Alkaline

One of the most important kinds of balance in the body is the acid and alkaline balance. Their characters are opposite and antagonistic. If they are mixed, they neutralize each other, but perfect balance is rare; one side is almost always stronger.

We know that the sour taste of lemons or vinegar comes from acid. To test this we can use litmus paper. If the blue litmus paper turns red, we have an acid taste or condition. The alkaline taste is not so easily identified, for we have no taste buds for this. Some call it bitter, but this is not accurate; probably a harsh soapy or potash taste is the expression of this taste. Alkali turns red litmus paper blue. We can taste acid or alkaline in foods, but when nutritionists say something is an acid food or an alkaline food, they don't mean this kind of testing by taste. After we eat a lemon and the body has absorbed or utilized it, the lemon leaves more alkaline elements than acid elements in the blood. Thus, the lemon is determined to be an alkaline-forming food and is sometimes referred to as an alkaline food. The taste of meat is not sour or soapy but is neutral in terms of acid and alkaline taste. However, after we eat meat and the body utilizes it, there are more acid elements left such as phosphorous and sulfur, and also the body produces uric acid from the purine bodies. Thus, meat is determined to be an acid-forming food and is sometimes referred to as an acid food.

Acid and alkaline depend on electric forces, both positive and negative. In solution, any substance that can donate a proton is an acid. An alkaline substance is one which can accept a proton. For convenience, it is common to express acidity and alkalinity by the hydrogen ion concentration and the resulting figure is called the pH. A pH of 7.0 is considered neutral; lower figures imply an acid solution and higher figures imply an alkaline one. A pH of 6.0 has ten times the hydrogen ion concentration than a pH of 7.0. A pH of 5.0 has one hundred times the hydrogen ion concentration and so on. In the same way, a pH of 8.0 has one-tenth the hydrogen ion concentration as a pH of 7.0. A pH of 14.0 is the strongest alkaline.

In a healthy body the pH of the blood is about 7.4, slightly on the alkaline side as compared to 7.0 in the natural world. The pH may differ slightly from person to person, but a range of 7.35 to 7.45 is considered a normal condition. Our body cells can survive only within this narrow range of the acid/alkaline balance. If this figure drops, we will suffer from acidosis and, if it goes below 6.9, we will go into a deeply unconscious state or coma, and possibly die. If the figure rises about 7.45, on the other hand, this is alkalosis; over 7.7 there can be active fits of muscular contraction and convulsion, which may also be fatal. Beyond these narrow limits we cannot live. Even a slight change in the blood pH makes for a big change in the state of our health. Therefore the body is always trying to keep the blood in a stable condition.

Homeostasis

The body needs to maintain an almost stable conditon in many areas. Some of these are body temperature, the total amount of blood and other body fluids, the proportion of glucose, protein, and all other nutrients in the blood, and the amount of oxygen. This concept is called homeostasis and is one of the most important concepts in biology. But this need for stability does not mean to never change. Everything is changing ceaselessly. The environment, food, activities, nothing is always the same. So, the body is constantly adjusting to any changes to form a new balance. This dynamic stability is the true homeostasis.

The quality of our blood is crucially important for the body cells, the body's 75 trillion citizens. The blood and circulating fluids create the internal environment. The cell's health and activities are entirely dependent on the quality of the blood. In the blood the acid/alkaline balance is especially important. Many organs are working for this balance – the kidneys, lungs, intestines, circulatory system, adrenal and pituitary glands; even the skin, muscles, and bones are all involved. Also, the body has a buffer system for sudden changes. The main factors effecting this balance are the foods we eat, the air we breathe, and our physical and mental activities.

Blood Acidity and Alkalinity

All foods can be determined as acid- or alkaline-forming. They vary in degree from strong acid-forming to almost neutral to strong alkaline-forming. Measuring a person's blood by examination is next to impossible because the test would have to be done only after eating one food and would have to be done at many time intervals. So, chemists examine acid and alkaline in a different way. The food is burnt and the ash is analyzed to determine the chemical elements that remain. Certain elements such as sodium, potassium, calcium, and magnesium carry a positive electrical charge (or $^+$ions) and have been determined to be alkaline-forming. Chlorine, phosphorous, and sulfur carry a negative electrical charge (or $^-$ion) and are determined to be acid-forming. The total amount of alkaline-forming elements that are left after burning are compared with the total amount of acid-forming elements and the food is then classified as to the degree of alkaline-forming or acid-forming ability. Still, this value can only be taken as approximate. Examples of this kind of analysis are shown in Table 15.

Reviewing this table, we can see that vegetables are in general all alkaline-forming foods, seaweed being the strongest, followed by cucumbers and tomatoes in the strong category; then the middle group – carrots, spinach, cabbage, and many varieties of fruit – and

Table 15. Acid- and Alkaline-Forming Foods[1]

Alkaline-Forming Foods			Acid-Forming Foods	
hijiki (seaweed)	65.00	(strong)	egg yolk	51.83
wakame (seaweed)	61.00		egg (whole)	24.47
green tea	53.50		chicken	24.31
cucumber	31.05		beef	22.95
tomato	13.67		lamb	20.30
sweet potato	10.31		cheese	17.49
turnip	10.18		sardine	17.35
orange	9.62		oatmeal	14.57
carrot	9.07		pork	12.47
grape	7.15		bread (white)	10.99
potato	6.71		walnuts	9.22
coffee	5.60		salmon	8.33
spinach	5.12		white flour	8.31
apricot	4.79		egg white	8.27
cabbage	4.02		chocolate	8.10
radish	3.06		margarine	7.31
black tea	3.04		ham	6.59
celery	2.05		bread (whole wheat)	6.13
watermelon	1.83			
mushroom	1.81	(weak)		

finally the weak alkaline foods such as celery and watermelon.

Eggs, chicken, and beef are strong acid-forming foods; cheese, sardines, and pork in the middle range; grains and nuts a little weaker; chocolate and margarine weaker still. In a processed food such as ham, the ratio is significantly changed due to added salt and other substances.

The components of foods will also vary according to the area where they are produced, the quality of the soil, and other factors. This problem is one of food composition analysis, but it is wise to understand which food groups are acid-forming and which are alkaline-forming.

Acid and alkaline neutralize each other and thus some food combinations are balanced with respect to acid and alkaline when eaten at the same meal.

Is Sugar Acid?

Once again, the question of sugar. Sugar itself is neutral, neither acidic nor alkaline, which seems good. But if we take sugar, it is absorbed and distributed to the body cells so quickly that sufficient supplies of oxygen are not yet readily available to burn the sugar completely. The incomplete burning that takes place produces lactic acid, pyro-racemic acid, butyric acid, acetic acid – all of them organic, but capable of creating acidosis in the body. For this reason sugar is an acid-forming food. Honey is said to contain alkalizing minerals that make it an alkali-forming food, but its metabolism by the body is the same as with sugar, so honey is actually an acid-forming food. Corn syrup, barley malt, maple sugar, and all other kinds of sweet concentrates are almost the same.

If we eat a starchy food such as potatoes or grains, the carbohydrates slowly turn to glucose and the smoky burning does not occur. So, there is no problem with the glucose level in the blood suddenly going up, even for a short time. This makes such a big difference.

Alkaline Foods Are Safer

Here is the problem. The body needs more acid-forming food than alkaline-forming food, so the body absorbs acid-forming food without limit. However, the small intestine only absorbs the amount of alkali-forming food that is needed. This sounds like a contradiction but is actually the body's protective mechanism at work. Body cells are weak against both sides, but in comparison they are stronger against acid and more sensitive to alkaline. Many kinds of microbes are stronger against acid than the body cells and weaker against alkaline. This means that we must limit the amount of acid-forming food we consume. This protective mechanism makes it easier to make balance. If we had no limit on either side, our life would be like tightrope walking; if we lose balance for even one second, we fall. With acid and alkaline, one side is dangerous but fortunately the other is safe. We don't run a double hazard.

To put it bluntly, acid-forming foods are dangerous and alkaline-forming foods are safe. This idea is not new. Early twentieth century scholars tried to teach us, but they received very strong opposition. The majority of nutritionists at the time believed another theory: that protein is the most important nutrient, that meat has the best quality of protein, and that the body needs meat. The scientists believed that if people quit eating meat because of the acid/alkaline theory, then the people would become malnourished, or deficient in protein. Many people were happy to eat meat because the taste is good. The acid/alkaline theory was not announced widely to the public.

Acid Blood Causes Trouble

Today many things are changing; heart trouble, kidney disease, etc., have greatly increased. Newly developed machines and techniques show that heavy meat-eating is harmful and that balanced nutrition is important. It is time to examine this acid/alkaline theory once more. Many kinds of diseases are related to acid blood.

Alkalosis never occurs when eating only natural food. If it should occur, it is always related to an overdose of chemical drugs such as bicarbonate of soda or a salicylate like aspirin. A few plants contain strong alkaloids and are poisonous; they are not food. The medicinal effects are well known and often used. Some examples are death-cup and other wild mushrooms, belladonna, and aconite (monk's hood). Such strong, concentrated alkaloids can pass through the intestinal walls and cause severe vomiting and diarrhea to eliminate toxins, but sometimes death can occur. These kinds of plants are excluded from the classification of natural food.

Alkalosis can be observed in other cases of severe vomiting or diarrhea, or if the patient loses too much potassium. But these troubles are already caused by acid blood. The best solution is to cut down on acid-forming foods such as meat.

Activity and Breathing

Another acid-forming factor is created by a deficiency of oxygen in the body. The body cells are always working and using oxygen. We continuously breathe and supply the blood with oxygen which is circulated throughout the body via the blood to all cells. Even a five-minute blockage of the windpipe can be fatal because the carbon dioxide which is produced as a metabolic waste of the cells is strong poison and must be carried off immediately.

Carbon dioxide is a gas. Hemoglobin in the blood can combine with oxygen but not with carbon dioxide. Carbon dioxide reacts with water molecules in the blood and forms carbonic acid. Larger amounts of carbon dioxide dissolve in water with the help of special enzymes and do not cause trouble. The blood carries both carbonic acid and carbon dioxide to the lungs where they are expelled from the body. Small amounts of carbonic acid are kept in the body for other uses.

We are always breathing and the body adjusts the amount of oxygen and carbon dioxide in the blood automatically. If the oxygen level goes down, we breathe more and increase the oxygen intake. If we use the body for heavy labor or for hard training, the cells use a lot of oxygen, the lungs become more active, breathing is deeper and more frequent, and the heart beats faster, sending more blood to the cells. But if not enough oxygen is supplied, carbonic acid accumulates in the body. The cells also make lactic acid, probably caused by the insufficient burning of fuel; lack of glucose and these acids cause fatigue. Under normal conditions the body recovers with rest or a good night's sleep. Even after extremely heavy physical work, the body returns to normal within a few days.

The Brain and Oxygen

The brain is the largest consumer of the oxygen in the body. The heart, lungs, and other organs are not as active when thinking or worrying as in the case of physical labor. Quite often they become more quiet and the body cannot get enough oxygen. For this reason, mental work is heavier labor than physical work and the fatigue can be much more severe. Mental stress is very strong. However, the brain is the smartest organ in the body and knows itself very well. If it is over-worked, it automatically begins sabotaging itself as I have written.

Almost everybody knows that if they take coffee, tea, or some drugs, they can stimulate the brain and force it to work continuously. Newly developed techniques such as positron emission tomography (PET) reveal brain cell activity with radioactively labeled glucose and show that the most active cells use the most glucose.[2] In this manner, if enough sugar is supplied, the brain can work more. But is this advisable?

Mental Stress

Forcing the brain to overwork can cause severe fatigue and the accumulated excess acid does not go away quickly. Insufficient burning of fuels caused by excess sugar and not enough oxygen produces other organic acids. Accumulation of these acids can cause brain damage and can leave the brain more susceptible to the attack of microbes. Alzheimer's disease, many encephalitic troubles, and other brain diseases are increasing in great number, much more so than a hundred years ago. Often it is said that mental stress causes diseases, but such stress is itself caused by overworking the brain supported by sugar and other stimulants. The true cause is always the same: excess acid in the body leads to many diseases.

In the normal, healthy body it is possible to become stronger and stronger for physical or mental work or even for stresses because the body reacts immediately and tries to recover quickly, carrying out excess acids. By taking in more alkaline elements, the body acquires a better ability to make balance. However, if the body becomes ill even once, this normal function does not work as well. In this case, clearly food is more important.

Acids produced by food metabolism are different. Phosphoric, sulfuric, and uric acids can only be excreted by the kidneys, so these acid-forming factors are important. The opposite opinion is that if we eat one pound of meat at one meal, blood tests do not show any abnormality. But this is on a daily basis. If you check many times a day, the protein content of the blood is always changing slightly. The buffer system is also working and chemical and protein buffers used should be replaced quickly. Once the blood test shows acidosis, it is often too late for a perfect recovery. Diabetes, kidney diseases, and lung disorders are said to be caused by acidosis, but actually the opposite is true. Acid blood causes these diseases first and then they become more severe as the excess acids remain in the blood.

Urine Acid Test

This is not an accurate test, but to get an approximate value of blood pH test paper (Nitrazine paper) is available at pharmacies. The quality of urine is not the same as that of the blood, of course, for the kidneys concentrate the waste products of cell metabolism and excrete them with the urine. Usually the urine pH shows a slightly higher value than the blood pH. The two main sources of acid are from food and from cellular activity. After heavy physical work, fatigue, or fever, more acids are excreted from the kidneys and your urine pH will test higher. But if your urine tests always reveal a higher degree of acid, then this is from your food, because the total input and output are always the same.

The normal pH of urine is considered to be between 6.3 and 6.6. But many Americans show a reading of about 5.3 to 5.6. This means that the ionized hydrogen concentration is about 10 times above the normal condition and clearly suggests too much acid-forming food. As long as the kidneys are maintaining normal functioning, they can handle this much acid. But it is possible to exceed the capacity of the kidneys, so this is a warning to you. You must reduce your acid-forming food intake and increase your alkaline-forming food consumption.

The Nitrazine paper test is best taken in the morning just after waking up, so try to test before eating or engaging in physical activities. In addition, it would be good to take the test many times a day, as urine tests show a wide range of fluctuation.

Body Control Mechanisms

The body's control mechanisms are mainly the nervous and hormonal systems. These are the body's balancing systems. Everyone knows about the sensory and motor nerves with which we control our physical activities, protecting ourselves from injury and controlled by our will power. But we know almost nothing about the activities of the internal organs or the quality of the blood. Everything is controlled by the autonomic nervous system, so usually we don't need to worry. We can will our lungs to breathe deeply, but most of the time the lungs and other organs are working without our consciousness.

The Autonomic Nervous System

The nervous system is a one-way communication. As part of the motor nerves, the autonomic nervous system has two components, sympathetic and parasympathetic systems, with opposing effects. They are connected to the brain through the hypothalamus and are totally controlled by the brain. They also have a connection to the pituitary gland. If the sympathetic nervous system is stimulated, the parasympathetic system becomes weaker, and vice versa. They interact by means of an on-off switch mechanism.

In emergency cases or sudden changes such as pain, rage, fright, anger, cold, exercise, ingestion of drugs, asphyxia, or other stress and physical activities (nearly all acid-forming factors in the blood), the sympathetic system responds by increasing the blood pressure, pulse rate, heartbeat, perspiration, and the blood sugar. It also activates the hypothalamus-pituitary system, leading to increased hormone secretions by the pituitary and adrenal-cortical steroid hormones in preparation for stress. When these emergency states have passed, the parasympathetic system overcomes the sympathetic and the body goes into a relaxed condition. At night, the parasympathetic system allows good sleep, as long as nothing stimulates the sympathetic system to wake up.

The parasympathetic system is concerned with the initiation and maintenance of a number of specific functions, such as digestion, intermediate metabolism of foods, and excretion. These activities are usually initiated in response to specific stimuli; a pleasant smell of food will create a relaxed condition and stimulate the appetite, or an erotic movie may serve to enhance the sex drive. If, however, any emergency arises during these pleasant conditions, the sympathetic system immediately responds; the parasympathetic system is overcome, the appetite is lost, and the body prepares for the urgency.

In general, the sympathetic nerves work for uses of energy while the parasympathetic nerves serve the body for resting and restoring of energy. Acids stimulate the sympathetic nerves, the cell metabolism becomes more active and produces more acid in the blood. But the sympathetic nerves hardly ever continue to dominate for a long time and if they do, fatigue or other strong reaction results.

Foods and the Autonomic Nerves

Whenever we consume coffee, alcoholic drinks, or foods that are too strong-tasting or -smelling, too hot or cold, or too spicy, the sympathetic nerves are stimulated. These are short-term reactions. Animal meats contain sodium, potassium, and other alkaline elements. Until it reaches the liver, meat creates work for the alkaline side. After it is utilized and produces sulfuric, phosphoric, and uric acids, the sympathetic nerves are stimulated causing hyperactivity, high blood pressure, fast pulse, higher body temperature, insomnia, and other abnormal conditions.

Vegetables, especially those often eaten raw, have a slightly acid taste which stimulates the sympathetic nerves slightly. But after they are absorbed into the bloodstream, potassium, calcium, and magnesium (which are all alkaline-forming) are activated so that strong reactions usually do not occur. However, vegetables do not contain much sodium or chlorine. These must be supplied from other sources.

Hormones

Another body-controlling system is the hormonal system. About twenty years ago only about twenty kinds of hormones were known. The endocrine gland was thought to produce all hormones, which were considered to be chemical messengers with special signs. The hormones were thought to be sent into the bloodstream and circulated until they reached an organ that understood the message and which then activated cells, produced more specific substances, or reduced activities or production.

Hormone research is much more advanced today. About two hundred kinds of hormones have been discovered. Not only specific glands, but also the kidneys, heart, liver, and many other organs, tissues, and even cells produce special substances to send messages to other organs, parts, or cells, and are all called hormones. The definition has become much wider. Especially exciting discoveries are that the brain also produces hormones and that at least forty-five separate hormones have been identified that control the whole body.

Every month new knowledge is added and hormone study has become complicated research. Only one rule is clear and always exists: if any hormone stimulates, another hormone of opposite character restrains. These opposite yet complementary hormones always work together along with the feedback systems to make good balance.

Hormones Work With the Nervous System

Many hormonal secretions are regulated by the autonomic nervous system through the hypothalamus and the pituitary gland. For example, the sympathetic system stimulates the hypothalamus to release a special hormone to the pituitary gland. The pituitary gland reacts immediately to release its own hormones (such as ACTH), which stimulate the adrenal cortex to secrete cortisone to increase blood sugar. More directly, the sympathetic system has a special relationship to the adrenal gland (medullary) cells and can release adrenaline (epinephrine) in the case of an emergency.

It is good to know a little about the hormonal feedback mechanisms. For example, the pancreas secretes insulin to regulate blood sugar. If the level of blood sugar goes up, the pancreas itself reacts to the higher blood sugar content and releases more insulin to reduce the sugar level, if everything is functioning normally. The pancreas also produces the hormone glucagon, which counteracts the insulin. Many other hormones also take part in the regulation of blood sugar.

The hormone researcher's dream seems to be to synthesize all kinds of hormones for use as medication to make the body taller, to lose weight, or to control any malfunction of the body or disease. For the normal, healthy person, the body produces all these hormones in a balanced way and hormones should not be added from the outside. This is different from nutrients such as vitamins and minerals which we have to take from food.

Foods and Hormones

We know only a few things about the relationship between food and hormones. One of them is the relationship of sugar and insulin. Another is between salt and aldosterone. The kidneys secrete the hormone renin to regulate the electrolytes and the water in the body. The adrenal cortex reacts to the renin and releases aldosterone. The kidneys then excrete more potassium and reabsorb more sodium, so we want to eat less salt. Other examples are that chewing increases secretion of the saliva hormone, parotin, and foods high in iodine such as seaweeds increase the thyroid hormone, thyroxine.

The relationship between food and many other important hormones including the sex hormones, androgen and estrogen, is not clear. But we do know that the central controlling mechanism is the brain. Many hormonal secretions are controlled by the brain through the autonomic nervous system and the relationship between food and the nervous system is becoming more clear.

Central Control

We have come to a basic point here: The brain controls everything through the nervous and hormonal systems. But what controls the brain? If anything can control the brain and the activities of the nervous system, it is the quality of the blood. The quality of the blood is controlled by the brain and the autonomic nervous system, but at the same time, food has a great influence on the quality of the blood, especially in regard to the electrolytes. And we can choose the quality of our food by our will power. Thus even the areas of human psychology, emotions, and behavior are related to food.

Once we understand this, the prevention of disease becomes much easier. And if we continue to maintain a good balance, the natural process of healing disease may even follow. We just need to pay attention to the foods we eat. The most important thing is maintaining the balance of the autonomic nervous system. For this purpose, the electrolyte or acid/alkaline balance is most helpful.

Malfunctions of the Nervous System

Next, you need to know the signs of a malfunctioning nervous system. Here are some examples as an introduction to the study of natural hygiene and dietary remedies.

Many people think of themselves as healthy or normal, but many of these people have one or more of the following problems. For sick people, probably the autonomic nervous system is already malfunctioning. If this is the case, just follow the dietary recommendations. The appearance of any of the signs mentioned in the rest of this chapter is the first stage of disease, and they need to be corrected as soon as possible. These indicate that your diet has been unbalanced for many years. The entire system of natural hygiene amounts to understanding the body as a whole and not as a combination of many parts like a machine. The human body is thousands of times more efficient than the most developed machines.

Sleeping Disorders

If you take more than ten minutes to fall asleep at night, wake up at midnight, have too many dreams, cannot wake up immediately in the morning, still feel sleepy in the morning, or if you sleep too long with shallow sleeping (except for children more than eight hours is too long), you are in the first stage of disease. In these cases, too many acid-forming foods have been consumed.

For such problems, don't take any sleeping pills or tranquilizers; try physical work or exercise. If you have no improvement, try more heavy exercise until you can sleep. For irregular sleeping reduce your meat consumption. Prolonged shallow sleeping or always feeling sleepy are caused by a shortage of electrolytes in the body. White sugar contains almost no electrolytes and white flour, white rice, and peeled vegetables have lost most of their important electrolytes, as have most refined and highly processed foods.

Another sleeping problem comes about because of midnight or overnight working. In modern society many companies want workers to work overnight. This disturbs the body's biological cycle and the rhythm of the autonomic nervous system. For at least a million years our ancestors slept at night and worked in the daytime and our bodies have completey adapted to this routine. But since the electric lamp was invented about a hundred years ago, nighttime working has increased. We cannot change so suddenly. For example, the temperature is usually lower at night and higher during the day and our body temperature also is higher in the daytime and lower at night, whether asleep or awake. This means our activity is slowed at night. Of course we can resist to a certain degree, but not perfectly. After many years of such living, some abnormal symptoms may appear. Probably impotence is one such kind of trouble. The incidence of impotence is higher among taxi drivers, many of whom are driving overnight and sleeping during the day. Of course there are other factors, but still the relationship seems undeniable.

Midnight eating or drinking is not healthy except if you must work at night. Do not eat later than two hours before going to bed.

Withstanding Cold

The problem of being too sensitive to cold or cold weather has a more important meaning. The abnormality is clear but the cause is perceived to be unknown. The cause is probably related to a sodium and calcium deficiency and with a lack of training. This condition also often indicates that serious diseases are at the root of the trouble, so it should be dealt with at this stage. Some people cannot touch tap water without it feeling like an electric shock. Even a room temperature of from 50°F to 60°F feels unendurable. If you catch cold easily or often in the summertime, this is also a warning signal.

If you cannot tolerate cold, training is needed. In the beginning, start to accustom your fingers to cold tap water or go out for a few minutes in the cold weather. Next, wash your hands and face with cold water. If possible, it is good to take cold showers or baths, even in the winter. But be careful not to catch a cold while doing any of these exercises.

Houses, cars, offices, etc., are heated so comfortably and hot water is available at any time; these are a credit to technology but also contribute to the deterioration of the human body. It has not yet been proven, but my opinion is that decreased sodium and excess potassium in the blood almost always contribute to this condition. By training the body to withstand the cold, it takes in and stores more mineral electrolytes, thus making the body warmer.

Sensory and Motor Nerve Disorders

Numbness, twitching, spasms, or cramps are signs of nervous

disorders and are directly related to the electrolytes, especially sodium, potassium, calcium, and chlorine. Slight cases are usually disregarded, but they shouldn't be.

Sugar removes many important minerals from the body, as I have already written. Therefore, all sensory and motor nerve disorders are related to eating excess sugar, and to a lesser extent excess coffee, tea, and drugs. Large doses of food supplements cannot compensate for this mineral loss. It is better to quit eating sugar.

Many health problems, including excessive sensitivity to cold, are related to sugar consumption to some degree. Sugar is the worst food humans have ever made. Now the world's sugar production exceeds more than 28 percent of all agricultural products; this makes the future of humanity look dark, but we do not need to follow what the majority of people are doing. Such disorders can be adjusted by controlling the intake of minerals (electrolytes).

Skin Trouble, Bad Posture, and Body Balance

Many skin problems such as dryness, oiliness, or sweating too much or too little during physical work are related to heavy meat-eating and also to improve chewing of food. They are also related to sugar-eating which you can discover for yourself by quitting the consumption of sugar.

Bad posture is similar in its cause. Excess acidity in the blood causes bad posture, which is accompanied by fatigue. Big shock for slight happenings, abnormal fear of animals, or other fears such as acrophobia are also signs of the early stages of disease.

Deterioration of the body's balancing mechanism is considered a sign of aging, but some people maintain a good balance into their seventies and eighties, while today some young people are losing theirs. Try these tests. Stand with your feet together and eyes shut. Keep your body straight for more than thirty seconds. Next, stand on your left leg and hold the big toe of your right foot with your left hand. Stand up straight and close your eyes for more than ten seconds. Repeat with the opposite foot and hand. If you have difficulty keeping a straight posture, you are losing the function of body balancing.

Many cases of motion sickness and the deterioration of the body's balancing mechanism are related to excess animal food eating. The high content of uric acid in the blood is one culprit. Ammonia, ketone, and other acids may be related also. A full stomach or stomach troubles makes one more sensitive to motion. Blood-alkalizing drugs such as Marezine can relieve the motion sickness temporarily but cannot stop the deterioration of the body's balancing function.

Not enough physical activity also encourages deterioration of the body's balancing mechanism, so always try to walk or do some physical work or exercise, especially if you have a sedentary job.

There are many more signs indicating the deterioration of good body balance and control, so please think of them yourself. For example, I did not list chronic fatigue, frequent fevers, weight loss, headaches, and many other conditions. These clearly indicate the early stages of disease, and some are the early symptoms of AIDS. In the next chapter, we will look carefully at some of these symptoms.

Chapter 16

AIDS Symptoms
and Strategies

With the many different opinions and kinds of information circulating in our society, there is much confusion. What causes AIDS? Is it a virus? What is the transmission route? How is the disease related to lifestyle? What about blood tests and other examinations? Many opinions have been established but nothing has been proven.

Another question is that of discrimination against people with AIDS. The newspapers, magazines, and books are full of stories about the sexual activities of AIDS patients. Margot J. Fromer wrote that "AIDS patients can have as much sex in as many different ways as they did before getting sick," and that one patient "admitted to having sex with 'dozens' of men since he had been diagnosed with AIDS." The patient "believes that AIDS is not contagious anymore anyway. If a prostitute who is infected quit her job, she cannot continue to support herself. And as long as she is 'feeling better' she will most likely continue her job."[1] Another author, Gene Antonio quotes Dr. John Dwyer, the former Chief of Immunology at Yale-New Haven Hospital, who treated more than four hundred AIDS patients: "Every now and then there are people who say, 'I know I'm going to die and I'm going to take as many people with me as I can.'"[2] If these cases seem to be abnormal or to indicate mental illness, that may be right. New research is showing that the AIDS virus can attack the brain cells directly before destroying the immune system. This is called AIDS encephalopathy (see Chapter 17).

If these kinds of stories were more widely known, then the healthy would be recommending the quarantine of AIDS patients and all virus carriers. The estimated number of carriers in this country is from two to three million. Considering how much money this would require, the government would of course say it was impossible to do. Then the big question is how to protect the healthy general public. During this difficult time a strange thing has happened. The FDA gave its official endorsement for the use of AZT (azidothimidine) for the medical treatment of AIDS. But reading the records of these tests we find that the patients feel better and the white blood cells increase only temporarily. This is not a permanent cure. And sometimes severe side-effects such as anemia have been seen.

In the past such drugs have only been allowed to be used for test cases. I thought the FDA and the Health Department existed mainly to protect the general public from disease. But this time it appears that the opposite has happened.

My original intension was to write only about AIDS prevention, but since the situation in the United States is so urgent, I have decided to write a little more.

Even though AIDS is considered terminal, there are always exceptions. If you have the right understanding and a strong will to live, even if you have full-blown AIDS, still you have a chance to recover perfectly. I am writing this chapter for sick people. Even though some of the material is repeated elsewhere in the book, if this helps you, then my effort is rewarded. Still, the strategy is limited to food only.

The Earliest Symptoms

In normally healthy people, the first stage of AIDS usually begins with slight symptoms similar to those of the common cold or the flu, but the illness is unclear. Care should be taken at this stage, for such slight symptoms can suggest that a serious disease is in the background. In many cases of AIDS it has been found that the initial symptoms resemble those often associated with the flu, but people pay little or no attention to them. Loss of appetite, fatigue, fever, and headache are seen very commonly. These are referred to as prodromes, or pre-AIDS symptoms, not sure signs of the disease, but possible indicators. If the disease advances, the next stage will include skin problems, coughing, night sweats, diarrhea, swollen lymph nodes, and other symptoms. If two or more of these symptoms accompany the above mentioned prodromes and no specific cause can be assigned, then it is possible that the person is infected with the AIDS virus. An antibody test will show a positive result, but the person will still not have all the symptoms of full-blown AIDS. These cases are called the AIDS-Related Complex (ARC).

Fatigue

If we were to look for the most common symptom in the earliest stage of many diseases, it would be fatigue. AIDS is no exception, so fatigue should be cured at this stage no matter the cause.

Everyone feels tired after using the muscles or brain. For heavy physical work the muscles need extra oxygen and glucose, the body temperature tends to go up, and, to regulate body temperature, sweat is released from the skin. The body loses water, salt, and other minerals. The muscles produce more lactic acid, which accumulates and causes fatigue. But the most important factor in the cause of fatigue is lack of oxygen. A sufficient supply of oxygen is crucially important in the prevention of fatigue, since the heart and lungs must increase the rates of circulation and respiration as the body becomes more active. As a result the lungs take in more oxygen and release it into the bloodstream. But this capacity for oxygen replenishment is limited. If we continue to use our muscles, the body cells will suffer an oxygen shortage and carbonic acid will be produced; this accumulates in the tissues and causes fatigue.

Oxygen is more important to the functioning of the brain than it is to the operation of the skeletal muscles. When we are using the brain, the lungs are not being activated – our breathing becomes shallower and, as we think or worry, we feel more tired.

The kinds of fatigue discussed here are all normal; if we take a rest or have a good night's sleep, it disappears quickly, within two to three days or a week at the most. In these cases, the cause of fatigue is clear and there is no need to worry about the presence of disease. Fatigue can protect the body from overuse of the muscles or brain. But if other symptoms accompany your fatigue, the situation is different. For example, if the urine is cloudy at the times of chronic fatigue, you most likely have kidney trouble and excess protein is being released. If the color of the urine is extremely dark, it may be due to hepatitis. Check your eyes: if they are yellow, this is a further indication; if the feces are whitish, then it is almost surely hepatitis or jaundice. If the urine smells like rotten fruit, it probably means diabetes. These are not the early signs of disease, but rather indications of more advanced stages.

Clearly, insufficient intake or excessive use of oxygen are the most important factors in producing fatigue. About twenty years ago on the streets of Paris, coin-operated machines dispensed oxygen, but such treatments discourage the body's own work. Even at high altitudes the body adjusts to the thin air and can become stronger by such training. There are other techniques for increasing oxygen in the blood.

Straighten Up Your Body

Observe your posture in a full-length mirror. If you have chronic fatigue your head will droop forward as in Figure 13(B). Try to hold your body straight, as in (A). In this position you can breathe deeply and take in more oxygen. Try to stay like this for the rest of the day. It is very difficult. Five minutes later you will notice your head drooping again. This condition is not easy to correct because it is a disease.

Figure 13. Posture

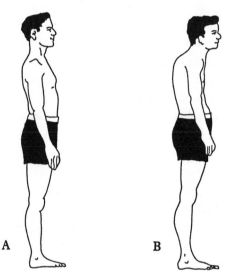

A   B

One experiment in adjusting this condition is to take a pinch of salt between the thumb and forefinger, probably about 0.3 grams or 5 grains of salt. Place it on your tongue for awhile without swallowing. The salivary glands react by secreting juices and the salt will dissolve. Now look in the mirror again. Within one minute your head will go into a straighter position by itself. Salt works before passing through the stomach and intestines; its beneficial effects are immediate. When the salt is dissolved and thinned out by your saliva and you no longer feel any irritation in your mouth, swallow it. This is not the best way to take salt, but to get quick results it may be used in this way like a drug. Usually, salt should be taken only with other foods in cooking or condiments.

After trying this experiment, if you find that ten or thirty minutes later your body is stooped over, try the same thing again. You can repeat it up to three times (that should be sufficient) but it is best to leave four or five hours or a day in between. Don't be in a hurry. Go slowly. Try it once in the morning and once in the afternoon, but it's not a good idea to do it at night. Excess salt can sometimes disturb a good night's sleep. In this experiment, don't take any additional liquids. Keep yourself slightly thirsty. If you wash out all the salt, no change may occur. After your body straightens, deep breathing becomes your normal condition, and you find that your fatigue is gone, don't take any more salt in this way. Use it only in your food.

What happens is that the sodium stimulates the parasympathetic autonomic nervous system, making the breathing slower and deeper and the heartbeat slower but more powerful. The chlorine helps the blood to carry away large amounts of carbon dioxide, helping to adjust poor posture and insufficient lung action. With the improved breathing you will notice increased movement of your abdomen.

If you feel bad after putting a pinch of salt in your mouth, spit it out. This means that your body already has enough salt and probably that your blood salt is the result of meat-eating. In this case probably your face, especially your ears, will look red. (A thin person seldom has this condition.) Then it would be a good idea to reduce your total food intake, eat raw vegetables to neutralize the acid in the blood and the excess salt, and avoid meat and sweet foods. The best foods for energy and regeneration at this point are small amounts of whole grains, which are high in thiamine (vitamin B_1) and provide a slow release of blood sugar, and foods high in calcium and dietary fiber such as dark leafy greens and sesame seeds. If available, sea vegetables are good.

Weight Loss

This is a common symptom of many different diseases; weight loss may also occur apart from disease, but that is another subject.

Generally speaking, the body loses weight during illness in an attempt to protect itself, especially among those who are overweight. In a larger body all the organs must work harder – the heart, kidneys, liver, lungs, and all the others without exception. With the increased volume of tissues in an overweight body, more blood is necessary to circulate and to clean, with more oxygen taken in and more hormones produced to adjust and control the various functions. For the white blood cells, always guarding the body against microbial or other agents of disease, a smaller area is easier to patrol than a larger one.

Unless you are extremely underweight, do not try to gain weight during sickness. Table 16 lists the optimum body weights for long distance runners, who often reduce their weight on purpose. For a man five feet tall, for example, the recommended weight is about 88 pounds; a man five feet, six inches should weigh about 115 pounds. These recommended weights are about 20 percent lower than the average figures, and I am assuming these as the optimal weight for fighting against disease-causing microbes. Even 30 percent lower than the average would be good.

It is best to trust your own body. Its 75 trillion body cells (including the white blood cells) all have the identical set of genes; they know everything about the body and can communicate with one another. Even if we fast for several days, our inner organs will not lose their vital powers. During a prolonged fast the body utilizes a process known as autolysis, meaning self-loosening or breaking down. The body burns and decomposes only excess fats or those tissues that are diseased, damaged, or of lesser importance to the body's economy such as abscesses.[3] The essential tissues of the vital organs are spared. The body knows and chooses exactly which tissues are most or least important.

In fasting, the eliminative and cleansing capacities of the lungs, kidneys, and skin are increased, in order to quickly expel the accumulated metabolic waste and toxic materials from autolysis. Breathing becomes deeper in order to oxygenate the blood, and the

Table 16. Runners' Weight Charts[4]

Height	Av.	-10%	-20%	Height	Av.	-10%	-20%
			Men's Weights				
5'0" (60")	110	99	88	5'9" (69")	160	144	128
5'1" (61")	116	104	93	5'10" (70")	165	149	132
5'2" (62")	121	109	97	5'11" (71")	171	154	137
5'3" (63")	127	114	101	6'0" (72")	176	159	141
5'4" (64")	132	119	106	6'1" (73")	182	164	145
5'5" (65")	138	124	110	6'2" (74")	186	168	149
5'6" (66")	143	129	115	6'3" (75")	192	173	153
5'7" (67")	149	134	119	6'4" (76")	197	178	158
5'8" (68")	154	139	123	6'5" (77")	203	182	162
			Women's Weights				
5'0"(60")	100	90	80	5'6"(66")	130	117	104
5'1"(61")	105	95	84	5'7"(67")	135	122	108
5'2"(62")	110	99	88	5'8"(68")	140	126	112
5'3"(63")	115	104	92	5'9"(69")	145	131	116
5'4"(64")	120	108	96	5'10"(70")	150	135	120
5'5"(65")	125	113	100	5'11"(71")	155	140	124

urine is darker, indicating more effective excretion of waste matter and excess acids; these are good signs that healing power is restoring the body. Fasting also stimulates the pituitary gland to release a growth hormone which activates the thymus gland to boost the body's immune response. Domestic pets and animals in the wild all use this same natural method of releasing healing power through fasting.

Eating with no appetite is a bad habit. Such excess nutrition only makes extra blood-cleansing work for the liver and kidneys and provides more acids as nutrition for unwanted microbes. The breathing becomes shallower due to a full stomach, oxygen intake is thus reduced, and the person is definitely fatigued. At such times I recommend taking only a vegetable broth. Simmer many different vegetables (celery, chard, mustard greens, carrots, potatoes, etc.)

in water for about half an hour and drink the broth only, without the vegetables. Your stomach will feel satisfied and the many minerals and vitamins in the broth will alkalize the blood. Don't eat until your appetite returns.

A ten- to twenty-pound weight loss is nothing to worry about for a 150-pound body. But I cannot say the same for those who are extremely thin to begin with; they have probably had a recurring problem for a long time. But this is not part of the early stages of illness, so I won't discuss it here. I can only suggest that underweight people chew well, two hundred times or more for each mouthful of food. It is true that you can chew your way back to a strong, healthy body.

Fever

Everyone has probably experienced many fevers as a part of the common cold, flu, measles, and other illnesses.

Fevers develop in many different ways. Sometimes the body temperature suddenly rises to 105°F or more and stays high for awhile; at other times, the temperature rises slowly, one or two degrees at a time over a period of several days, until it reaches a high temperature. Some fevers move up and down four or five degrees, others will appear every other day or once every three days. Atypical or irregular fevers are very common. There are also low fevers in which the body temperature rises slowly and remains one or two degrees higher than normal. The temperature is usually normal in the morning and rises in the afternoon, and this repeats for a few days. This is not necessarily bad, but if low fevers continue for many days it may indicate that a serious disease is behind it.

Unusually high or long-lasting fevers are neither desirable nor comfortable and are to be avoided if possible. Sometimes fevers are life-threatening; it is said that a temperature above 108°F can cause brain damage. So the questions are: Why do we have fevers, what do they mean, and how should we handle them? Current research on these questions has brought some changes in medical thought.

Most of the body's enzymes are inactive at low temperatures and are also destroyed by high temperatures. Our body enzymes work best at about 103°F to 104°F. For quick movement of our muscles and for active movements of the organs, a higher body temperature is a great advantage, so all developed animals have higher body temperatures. The most active animals are the birds that fly and they have the highest temperatures. For their activities, warm-bodied animals consume more food for fuel; this can be one of the disadvantages of a warm body. The heat of a body is the balance between heat gained and heat lost.

The Body Needs Fever

High fever activates the whole body: The heart beats more; the lungs breathe more frequently; the liver increases its activity, destroying more protein and fat; the kidneys excrete more acids in order to clean the blood. The endocrine glands produce more hormones in order to maintain normal functions of the body, and the body cells produce more interferons and interleukins to fight against disease.

For physical activities, a slightly higher temperature is desirable; for mental activities, a little lower temperature seems better.

For the past hundred years the treatments prescribed for fever were always intended to lower the fever as quickly as possible through the use of aspirin and other anti-fever drugs. Ice bags, ice caps, and ice pillows were used for cooling the body so that the patient would feel more comfortable. Recent discoveries show that these treatments were almost always inappropriate. Fever is the body's natural defense mechanism. It inhibits the growth and activity of microbes, often destroying them; therefore, it is best to let a fever run its course. The temperature will come down on its own. When ice treatments are applied to the fevers of measles patients, complications often result. By failed experiments it was finally learned that cold water or ice should not be used for measles; just stay in bed in a warm room and let the fever go up. Measles is not such a dangerous disease; 99 percent of all patients have a nice recovery without any special treatments at all. Most people were already aware of this even prior to the development of vaccines. Only in those rare cases in which the temperature exceeds 106°F will some kind of protection be needed against damage to the brain.

Fever indicates that the fuel (carbohydrates) in the body are burning too fast. This is why through fever the body loses weight. But in many cases, fat and protein are destroyed and burned as fuel; almost one pound of protein can be destroyed in a day. I believe this is excess or poor quality protein that the body wants to get rid of. Before unwanted microbes can absorb this excess nutrition, fever is used as a weapon to burn up the fuel. Clearly, it is a mistake or maltreatment to give a high protein diet in an attempt to prevent weight loss when there is a fever. Eggs and chicken, commonly recommended foods for sick people, are actually the worst foods for the sick as these are high octane fuels in the human body. All red meats are dangerous foods for someone with a fever. Fish are cool-blooded, about 75°F, a little higher than the water they live in, so eating fish is not as harmful to a fever as poultry and other meats. But compared to plant foods, fish is still a high octane fuel for humans. If a person with a fever has an appetite, the best foods are vegetables, vegetable broth as described on pages 267 and 268, or bean protein. If there is no appetite, it is best not to eat. If you feel thirsty, warm water or warm tea is recommended. Mushrooms, slightly sour green apples, and raw radishes are often effective against a high fever.

In Case of Emergency

For extremely high or dangerous fevers, certain Asian treatments such as tofu plasters or carp blood and plasters are highly effective. These are excellent treatments to remember.

The best food for reducing a high fever is carp blood. It might seem strange that I would suggest an animal food as a cure, but carp blood has been an important traditional remedy in Asian countries for many years. Buy a live carp (Asian variety) from an Oriental market. The carp should be about ten to twelve inches long. Make a cut in the area of the snout with a large knife and hang the fish up. Catch the blood that drips out into a small glass. About one or two tablespoons of this blood is good enough; give it to the patient and within ten minutes the fever will have dropped by at least 2°F. Carp blood has a strong healing power and will not cause dangerous side effects.

If the fever is still high, though it has dropped several degrees, chop up the meat of the carp into small pieces and make a plaster which should be applied to the forehead, the back of the neck, and, if there is enough, to the chest. The temperature will drop quickly. Be sure to keep checking the temperature and when it reaches 100°F, remove all the plasters. If the temperature should drop below normal (about 98.6°F), it would be difficult to bring it up again and the patient may suffer terrible chills.

This carp treatment is not only marvelous for reducing fever but has other healing benefits as well, although these have not yet been established scientifically.

The only difficulty with this remedy is that carp is not always readily available. You can often find them in Chinese markets, but not always. If not, try to locate a carp fish farm. There are some carp farms which for economic reasons raise a German carp since the German carp grows faster than the Asian variety. The Asian carp (called the "Chinese grass carp") is preferable for this purpose, but, if you can't get it, the German carp will do.

If carp is not available, a tofu plaster can be used in its place. Just apply tofu to the forehead and the back of the neck. Tofu plaster also has this ability to reduce a fever and has other healing qualities.

Tofu is also called "soy cake" (or bean curd) and is readily available in supermarkets or Oriental food stores. The main component of tofu is soybean protein. Tofu may also be eaten, but as a food seems to have no special effect in lowering the body's temperature. But at the same time eating tofu seems to have no adverse effects either on a high fever or a weakened kidney condition. As with the carp remedy, make sure the temperature does not become too low.

Malaria

From ancient times and still now, the greatest killer of humanity is said to be malaria; it is the champion of fever diseases, so I will discuss this a little and we can learn many things.

All over the world today, including the United States, Canada, Northern Europe, and Russia, many people are affected by malaria, but in African countries malaria is most prevalent. In Africa alone about a million people die every year, and in India, Southeast Asia, New Guinea, and the other Pacific islands a billion people live under its constant threat. In ancient times this was almost exclusively a tropical disease, but the early Greeks and Romans did have malaria, so at that time the disease had already spread from the Far East to the Mediterranean, although it was not found in other areas of Europe until the end of the eighteenth century, when it reached epidemic proportions. It was widespread in North America by the middle of the seventeenth century, but has declined with the development of medicine and pest control. However, 1,056 cases were reported in the United States in 1982, many of these the most virulent forms of malaria, in spite of so much effort to control.

Malaria is caused by a kind of parasitic protozoa carried by mosquitoes from human to human. The parasites enter the red blood globules, destroy the host globules, and produce toxic substances. The body produces a high fever to kill them but some survive, reproduce within forty to sixty-four hours, and attack again. The body heats up again in its attempt to kill the parasites. The fever lasts about six to eight hours before the temperature returns to normal. If we try to stop the fever, this may involuntarily lead to a fatality.

The classic symptom of malaria is intermittent fever with chills and sweating. Half of the world's malaria is called tertian fever, with fever at intervals of forty-eight hours. Quartan malaria brings on chills and fever every seventy-two hours. Tertian fever is a benign form of the disease and is less formidable. A more virulent form of malaria called falciparum or pernicious malaria appeared later. The interval of this fever is about two days, but not so regularly. The fever may reach up to 107°F or more; 90 percent of the deaths which occur from malaria are associated with this form. An even more severe form of malaria has increased in this century, caused by the same type of parasites. The fever is irregular, large amounts of red blood cells are destroyed, and acute renal failure is accompanied by the passing of reddish-black urine. This dreaded complication is known as the blackwater fever, which is considered incurable.

The history of the spread of malaria clearly shows that the parasites invaded the North from the South, but evidence also indicates that northern peoples imported co-factors of malaria from tropical countries through the importation of tropical fruits, sugar, and much more. Those who did not eat much tropical food did not get malaria. Some examples are the people of the Pripet marsh region of Russia and the areas of Yaroslav and Kasan and others; people from the north of France; and those who lived on the northern and western islands of Britain. The Spanish were especially resistant to malaria and were thus able to spread over the world. All of these peoples were mainly grain-eaters.

The best medicine for controlling malaria was found to be quinine, originally a Peruvian folk remedy, made from the bark of the cinchona tree. With the synthetic medications for malaria that have been developed in this century, quinine has almost been forgotten. However, quinine may still be a good treatment for the control of fevers, not only for malaria but for many kinds of infections; it has no bad side effects, for it is a natural organic product. Among African AIDS patients with malaria, it might be worthwhile to experiment with quinine as treatment for the malaria fevers, which may be able to kill the AIDS virus. Very careful observation would be needed, along with dietary reconstruction of the immune system.

Fever Therapy

For centuries syphilis was such a difficult disease to cure, but when some patients were infected by other pathogenic germs involving high fever, they recovered from syphilis mysteriously. Doctors experimented with high fevers, heating the patient's body or exposing it to another disease, but fever therapy is obviously a risky treatment. In this century, when malaria and typhoid fever came under control, there were many such experimental tests; the University of Virginia Hospital has records of many successful treatments in the early 1940s.

Whether this kind of treatment can be used for AIDS or not is unknown as yet. To develop this idea, it would be necessary to go to tropical Africa and watch very carefully how malaria and AIDS work together.

Night Sweating

Sweating is well controlled by the body, for it is the principal method of body temperature regulation. Under normal healthy conditions, about one quart of water evaporates from the 2.5 million sweat glands every day. This involuntary action is called insensible perspiration. During sleep about a cup of water is evaporated from a healthy body. When we are active, the body temperature increases and we produce extra sweat in order to cool it down, but often excess sweat, or sensible perspiration, is produced. If during sleep the body produces sensible perspiration, this is called bed sweating or night sweating.

Even healthy people sometimes have night sweating. If, for example, we drink too much water, tea, alcohol, or other liquid, the body may excrete the excess through the skin. Another cause is the excessive intake of animal foods; the body craves liquids, the kidneys are overloaded with acids produced as a reaction, and the skin helps by excreting some of the acids through perspiration. In this case the sweat will normally test acid. This condition is also considered an imbalance of protein versus glucose in the blood, often controlled just by taking a few candies or other sweets after dinner. However, if bed sweating continues for several days, we have to think some kind of disease is behind this. Many kinds of fever can cause sweating, and this lowers the body temperature. Profuse sweating was often observed in malaria or rickets patients, and tuberculosis patients often had prolonged night sweats over a period of many years. Other respiratory disorders also often caused bed sweating.

For those who are in the high risk category for AIDS, persistent bed sweating may be considered as one of the symptoms of ARC. This is not a clear sign of AIDS, like Kaposi's sarcoma or PCP with immuno-suppression, but it is possible to fall into full-blown AIDS. This symptom suggests that the body still has strong resistance to disease, but that the respiratory system is already being affected by a virus or bacteria. AIDS is now often appearing with tuberculosis, especially in Haiti and Africa.

In these cases, the respiratory systems have been weakened by the excess consumption of sweets and sugar over many years; taking a few candies cannot control this bed sweating and would only make it worse. Over the years, sugar has removed calcium and other minerals, vitamin D, and other vitamins and protein. If the phosphorus ion (-) increases, the calcium ion (+) decreases in the blood and the kidneys excrete more calcium. To recover from such a condition is a slow and difficult process. Only good foods, especially those rich in calcium and vitamins B_1 and D, should be eaten. Avoid high phosphorous content foods such as cocoa, beef, pork, lamb, cheese, and poultry. I don't oppose calcium or vitamin B injections, but their good effects do not seem to last long.

Certain special foods can be useful in such cases; garlic is the most commonly available. The ancient Romans and Chinese believed that garlic is good for loss of appetite, respiratory disorders, leprosy, and other diseases. Recent scientific research has discovered that the medicinal effect of garlic comes from the elements it contains – germanium, allicin, adenosine, and others. Onions, scallions, chives, and leeks are in the same family and have similar good effects, reaching the lungs through the sense of smell. Choose a strong smelling garlic. Ginger, horseradish, mint, parsley, cinnamon, and many other plants are also beneficial. Even flowers, if they have a strong odor, probably have healing power. Keep them by your bedside or in the living room; they are not only beautiful, but it is good to breathe their fragrant smells.

Coughing

A cough is a violent expulsion of air following deep inspiration along with closure of the glottis. If any foreign substance or mucus causes an obstruction in the bronchial tubes, the body protects itself by removing it from the respiratory passages. This is a normal function in healthy people.

Some coughs are a result of allergies; some are caused by cardiac asthma or various other diseases. In these cases the causes of coughing are easily identified. But when healthy people start coughing for unknown reasons and it persists for a number of days with no cold or flu symptoms, it often indicates a serious disorder of the respiratory system.

In the bronchi a small amount of mucus is needed to protect the surfaces of the air tubes, but excess amounts are often produced, usually from heavy protein intake. This is needless protein for the body, so it is quickly discharged as mucus; however, in advanced respiratory illness, even important proteins can be lost in this way. The asthmatic cough occurs most often in the middle of the night and is often associated with meat-eaters; in the past, this was treated (except in cases of cardiac asthma) by taking much liquid to produce a sweat, or holding a candy in the mouth to give moisture to the throat. Ephedra, a wild desert plant from which the drug ephedrine is extracted, has often been a successful component in an herbal tea mixture, but must be used carefully as it can overstimulate weak people.

With colds or the flu, especially among the overweight, the bronchi may enlarge and swell up; large amounts of thick mucus are excreted, sometimes with blood, and the cough is similar to that associated with chronic bronchiectasis. For this condition, reduce all your food. These severe coughs and mucus discharges usually occur in the morning. Sweet food lovers and diabetics often have this kind of cough, which is opposite in character to the asthmatic cough. This is indicated by the doctor's treatment: adrenal hormones, adrenalin for the first type, and cortisone for the latter type. We can see that the first type of cough is associated with meat-eating and the second with the consumption of sugar. Dairy products also seem to produce more mucus and should be avoided.

Still another type of cough can be seen in cases of pulmonary tuberculosis. This is a weak cough. Its onset is unclear – it slowly creeps in and often the patient doesn't recognize it, as there is no great suffering. This cough is caused by excess sugar consumption and often leads to irreversible bronchiectasis. A small amount of blood along with mucus often appears from the trachia, the bronchia, then the lungs. The body appears to be exhausted from malnutrition, so good nutrition and intake of salt are important. Sauteed grains and vegetables with sesame oil and salt is a good way to take salt. Check your palm to monitor fat deposits before using oil, as described in the chapter on animal foods.

Haitian and African AIDS patients often have tuberculosis, and in this country also it is making a dramatic comeback due to AIDS. Some researchers speculate that TB may actually cause immunosuppression and AIDS. This hypothesis has not been proven but much attention should be paid to anyone starting a weak cough as TB is highly contagious. Dr. Dixie Snider, Jr., of the Centers for Disease Control has warned that it is important that TB be diagnosed accurately. But unfortunately, now a strange thing is happening with the tuberculin skin test, long considered reliable in the diagnosis of tuberculosis: some people who have TB are not reacting to the test. Especially in AIDS patients, the skin test is almost always negative, but they are dying of TB as a secondary infection. Because the immune system is already depressed, accurate diagnosis is difficult. Then the most important questions are, does the body look exhausted or does it appear to be receiving and utilizing sufficient nutrition? Other early symptoms of TB are fatigue, weight loss, low-grade afternoon fever, night sweats, shortness of breath, etc., but recently more atypical TB is increasing.

Retinachoroiditis (Cloudy Vision)

One of the ARCs is said to be retinachoroiditis, an inflammation of the retina and choroid in the deep part of the eye. This is not a life-threatening condition but it can be very frightening, especially with sudden onset. The inflammation may go away, but the vision deteriorates and floating objects resembling mosquitoes or other small flying insects appear before the eyes. Carefully observed, they look like spots or threads. The patient may try to brush them away, but the trouble lies within the vitreous humor of the eye and not on the surface. As these floating objects increase, the vision grows cloudy; the condition worsens each time the eyes become inflamed, so that the cloudy vision grows progressively worse. Finally the increased spots and threads connect with one another and the whole field of vision becomes cloudy and one is unable to see. Formerly this condition was reported in cases of syphilis, leprosy, and tuberculosis and later, with malaria, diabetes, and high blood pressure. But in recent years it has become quite common apart from these diseases; excessive meat and sugar consumption may encourage inflammation and the resulting cloudiness of vision.

Next to brain damage, this is one of the hardest conditions to remedy. No effective treatment has been found; it is considered a success if the progressing condition is controlled. If the floating images become mobile and the vision is disturbed, the condition is progressing; if they become less mobile and the threads shrink back to spots, this is a sign that your overall condition is improving. The process can be slow, and it seems that many people just give up. Statistical research says that about 30 percent of Americans have this deterioration; this is an unbelievably high number. This condition is very unfortunate, but you can use it as your health barometer. You may notice that even one piece of cake or candy can disturb your vision. Good weather or physical activities may seem helpful, while reading, overeating, too much sun, or too much thinking may make it worse. You can check foods one by one and classify the exact effects. This gives you a special ability in monitoring your health. But in the case of AIDS-related problems, this condition becomes quickly worse and you have no time to test. Quit eating meat and sugar immediately and prevent retina inflammation.

Diarrhea

As an early stage of disease, diarrhea is caused most commonly by overeating, undigested foods, and taking cold foods such as ice cream, ice water, cold beer, and other iced or frozen food and drink. When cold foods enter the stomach, the bottom gate, the pylorus, opens automatically and much of the contents of the stomach enter the duodenum whether or not they are fully digested. This is the cause of diarrhea for many Americans. People are paying money to buy diarrhea. Poor quality foods can also cause diarrhea, and in some cases there is food poisoning when toxic substances are taken by accident or mistake. In all such cases the body's defense mechanism is working properly by rejecting absorption and quickly eliminating these foods.

Other cases of acute diarrhea can be caused by contaminated water or food, as with dysentry or typhus, but these diseases are now well controlled in developed countries and seldom occur. There are also many diseases that can cause diarrhea – stomach or intestinal troubles, hepatitis, peritonitis, intestinal worms; even flu, pneumonia, measles, and smallpox often create this condition, but these cases are not under discussion here.

If normally healthy people have diarrhea, some kind of food has stimulated the colon excessively, perhaps an excess of fiber, although if we are eating natural foods it is almost impossible for this to occur. Undigested or badly-fermented food overstimulates the intestine, and this is mostly related to insufficient chewing (see Chapter 9).

Diarrhea is the frequent evacuation of residual food wastes from the bowel with much moisture and liquid. Two factors are clearly indicated: the large intestine is overactive, and there is too much fluid in the body; more cannot be absorbed. This probably indicates there is not enough salt in the body.

Watery stools are caused by an excessive intake of water or by the malabsorption of water by the intestines. The basic cause of this excessive fluid intake is the eating of highly concentrated foods, such as sugar, candies, strong alcohol or coffee, vinegar, animal meat, spicies, and overly salty foods such as corn chips or hot dogs. The body craves liquids in order to dilute these concentrated foods, but the taste of fruit juices or soft drinks is too good and it is easy to drink more than necessary. The underlying cause of the malabsorption of water is an insufficiency of good salt in the food or in the body, especially for those restricting their intake of salt. This deficiency can lead to chronic diarrhea.

From this condition, more complicated and chronic intestinal problems may begin. If many essential intestinal bacteria are lost through diarrhea, the digestion of food is not completed by the colon. Imbalances of the intestinal flora or insufficient bacteria in the colon may also be caused by the use of antibiotics that were prescribed for other infections. A healthy colon hosts more than four hundred varieties of bacteria, viruses, fungi, and other microbes, most of which are anaerobic – living without the need for oxygen.

The intestinal microbes maintain a delicate symbiotic balance with the body, and each species must also hold its place with all the other varieties. If this balance is lost or antibiotics are used, some species will die, others will increase, or the total number may decrease; the result is chronic intestinal trouble. Fortunately, if in the early stages of this deterioration our nutrition is basically good and the intestinal environment improves, the lost microbes can regenerate quickly. However, highly synthetic or chemicalized foods or foods containing preservatives cannot be a good culture for friendly microbes. Taking high doses of vitamins also disturbs the proper balance of the colonic flora.

Some Special Foods for Diarrhea

A good natural food remedy for diarrhea is kuzu (or kudzu) cream, taken over a period of several days. Three tablespoons of kuzu starch are mixed with two cups of cold water and simmered for about five minutes until it is creamy and looks translucent, and seasoned with ume juice (the liquid in umeboshi, Japanese pickled plums) or, as a second choice, natural soy sauce. This is taken in place of a meal. Kuzu is an important medicinal herb in Asian countries. The starch is extracted during winter from the kuzu root which actually grows everywhere in the southeastern United States. If kuzu powder is not available at your natural food store, thin creams of rice, oats, potato starch, or other starchy grains prepared with natural salt can be effective. Salt always seems to be an important part of the remedy for many kinds of diarrhea.

For diarrhea of an unknown cause or if it accompanies early AIDS symptoms, it may be good to try to take a little more salt. The well-known Dr. Tatsuichiro Akizuki, director of St. Francis Hospital in Nagasaki, Japan, discovered this just after the atomic explosion, centered less than a mile from the hospital. Akizuki observed bleeding and diarrhea in himself and many of his patients and, without knowing the cause (or the effects of radiation, nothing of which was yet written in medical books), made a salt solution a little more saline than blood serum. He found this very effective, and he also recommended that all his patients and staff take slightly salty miso soup every day and avoid sugar completely. He said sugar would destroy the blood. Even though Akizuki's hospital was much closer to the blast than the University Hospital, where 3,000 patients suffered greatly from leukemia, many of his patients recovered from the diarrhea and all of them were safe from radiation. Residents of Nagasaki called this a miracle.[5]

Under Akizuki's direction the hospital kitchen served brown rice, miso soup with a small amount of vegetables and seaweeds, rice balls with umeboshi plums, and that's all. No other foods were available and were not needed anyway according to Akizuki. My dietary recommendations are much wider and easier to take.

Chapter 17

Full-Blown AIDS

AIDS Encephalopathy

Researchers recognized early that many AIDS patients had mental and nervous system disorders, but it was not clear at that time what caused these problems. It was thought that perhaps the cytomegalovirus or the cryptococcus fungus were the culprits. But soon after HIV-I was identified as the AIDS virus, they were able through autopsies to detect the presence of the same virus in the brains and nervous systems of AIDS patients. So it soon became clear that the AIDS virus affects more than the immune system – that it directly attacks the brain and nervous system before destroying the immune system.

Only One Thing to Try

We learned from experience with rabies that once the rabies virus invades the brain cells, nothing can be done for the disease. The virus must be killed or inhibited from moving to the brain. Presumably the AIDS virus moves more slowly than the rabies virus. Therefore, we probably have enough time to prevent its reaching the brain. The problem is that it is not always clear when the patient is exposed to the AIDS virus. Also it takes longer to move from the genital area to the brain than from the mouth. Take advantage of this longer period. Change your diet and the virus may still be prevented from entering the brain. Even if an effective vaccine or drug were made and available today, after the virus reaches the brain cells, it would be too late. Remember that brain damage is mainly caused by the excess consumption of sweet foods.

And so the one thing you can do, starting today, is to change your diet to alkalize your blood and regenerate a strong immune system. Whether or not you are exposed to the virus or even infected doesn't really matter. The rules of prevention are the same in either case. Nothing else can really help.

Kaposi's Sarcoma

About 90 percent of AIDS patients have had Kaposi's sarcoma or *Pneumocystis carinii* pneumonia and some have had both. Kaposi's sarcoma is one of the clearest signs of the presence of AIDS. About 30 percent of all recorded AIDS cases have had Kaposi's sarcoma.

At the time Moriz Kaposi first described this disorder in 1872, microbes were not considered to be the cause of any infectious diseases. Following Kaposi's description, a rare and unusual tumor appeared both in Europe and America, but it took a more benign and indolent form. In these cases the victims usually survived anywhere from eight to twenty years following diagnosis and, because by that time so many of them were along in years, a number died of causes other than Kaposi's sarcoma.

The Kaposi's sarcoma associated with AIDS has been found almost exclusively among young men between the ages of twenty to sixty, the median age being about thirty-five. The appearance of this disease seems much different from what Kaposi described. Often, several or many spots or bumps of various colors appear suddenly. These tumors increase quickly and grow rapidly to form large-sized plaques. Although many cases originate on the legs or feet, others start from various parts of the body such as the mouth, genitals, hands, nose, etc. The plaque lesions are characterized by an increased number of jagged, irregularly shaped vascular spaces along with newly-formed capillary blood vessels full of red blood cells. Along these blood vessels are increased numbers of grouped, spindle-shaped cells located between the collagen bundles. The sarcoma can also grow in the gastrointestinal tract or in various organs.

Is KS a Cancer?

Scientists differ as to whether Kaposi's sarcoma is a cancer. For thousands of years our ancestors have had cancer, but it was never considered a contagious or infectious disease. The National Cancer Institute as late as 1979 stated in their literature that "scientists have found that cancer is not contagious" and that "cancer is not transmitted to a sexual partner by sexual intercourse." In 1979 the first AIDS case was discovered and a few years later (1981) Kaposi's sarcoma was determined by some researchers to be a form of cancer.

Since everything in this world is constantly changing, I am not surprised by this change, but it can be frightening for the general public. During the past several hundred years cancer has been classified as a carcinoma and as a sarcoma. Historically, carcinoma has been referred to as a malignancy. Although it took a heavy toll on life, it was usually slow-growing and it was not unusual for patients to live for ten, twenty, or even thirty years following diagnosis. Often carcinoma patients died from other complications not directly related to the cancer itself. Carcinomas were recognized as neoplasms that occur on the skin, in the tissue lining of the body, or in the organs. They often metastasize (spread) to other areas of the body. At first, one or several cells develop an abnormality in the genes. The abnormal cell then duplicates itself and begins to multiply without limit. After many years of replication, a tumor is recognized.

Sarcomas were considered to be benign tumors, remaining localized in those areas where they first originated. Sarcomas rarely metastasized and normally appeared in the muscles, connective tissue, or bones. Over time, other cancers have made their appearance, including leukemia and lymphomas.

As early as 1910, Peyton Rous reported a form of cancer found in chickens that was caused by a virus and which was transmissible. This was the first record of an infectious cancer, but his discoveries were ignored and neglected by medical scientists. Fifty-six years later Rous was awarded the Nobel Prize. Now known as Rous Sarcoma, it is certain that some kinds of animal cancers are caused by virus and are contagious. Recent genetic research has shown that retroviruses enter the genes of the host cells and alter the genetic structure of those cells, which become abnormal and start to multiply without limit. This kind of retrovirus is called an oncogenic virus. Some DNA viruses have this same ability of unlimited proliferation. The role of viruses as a cause of cancer is now beyond question.

It is not clear what kind of virus alters the genes in the case of AIDS-related Kaposi's sarcoma. Since HIV-I has no cancer-forming ability and if Kaposi's sarcoma is considered a cancer, then cytomegalovirus or some other virus must affect the genes. The AIDS Kaposi's sarcoma tumor is not a metastasizing growth, but is multicentric, which means that the tumor can arise anywhere on the skin or within the body independently of the original tumor. Thus, some researchers claim that AIDS-related Kaposi's sarcoma is not cancer.

If a single causative agent of KS were discovered, then it would be easily treatable. Chemotherapy, radiation, and surgery have been the traditional medical treatments for cancer, but in many cases these treatments have failed to cure the disease. Through chemotherapy the primary cancer will often appear to have receded, only to be soon replaced by new, secondary cancers. Radiation and surgery often result in suffering and disability for the patient.

For treatments, Hippocrates reminded us that "the occult

growth was to be left alone, since the patient would live longer with the disease untouched." It has been estimated that two million Americans have not been cured of their cancers but are learning to live with them; some of these cancers are in remission, and some are progressing slowly or have not progressed far enough to be disabling or fatal.[1]

AIDS-related KS cannot just be left alone, for it progresses rapidly. In my opinion, KS is probably not a cancer, but whether it is or not is beside the point. There are many other kinds of fast-growing diseases that are also capable of a rapid cure. Burkitt's lymphoma, for example, is said to be a kind of cancer. It is sometimes found in African children manifesting as a fast-growing, mump-like tumor. If these patients get proper treatment in time, the tumor diminishes quickly. In California one doctor is treating AIDS-related KS by vitamin C therapy with some success. In the classic American form of KS, tumors are often found to disappear once the immuno-suppressive medications are discontinued.

Don't Eat Meat

Kaposi's sarcoma is probably one of the easiest to cure among AIDS-related infections. It is essential to stop eating meat and all other animal foods. Many diseases caused by excess meat-eating follow a quick progression and a quick recovery. Heavy meat-eaters are easily prone to infections but are capable of an easier recovery than those who fall ill from eating an excess of plant foods.

Protein and sugar are the most important nutrition for microbes. To stop eating meat is a kind of starvation strategy. Don't give nutrition to your enemy. You may feel a little hungry, but the microbes' situation becomes much worse. Even if you lose one million body cells, if you can kill one million enemies, you can win this battle. Remember, you have 75 trillion body cells.

In many cases the tumors shrink within three months, but this does not mean they are completely cured. You have to stick to a vegetarian diet until the tumors and lesions are completely healed.

Do not eat animal food, especially red meat, until your medical tests show that your body has produced enough antibodies and white blood cells. In the cases of malignancies, relapses have been seen within two days after the patient ate meat. Why does such a sudden change occur? Most likely because the cells have not changed. In cases of carcinoma, about seven years are needed for a change of cells. Kaposi's sarcoma is a different story but still it may take from one to three years. Until all abnormal cells have changed to normal a patient has not recovered.

A problem occurs when people remember all the palatable food they enjoyed in the past and begin to crave them. To not eat any more meat and sugar is easy to say. But we live in a strange world; some people want to eat meat even if it costs them their lives. Something is beyond our minds, some will or unconscious intention, maybe from genetic memory.

Another common reason for returning to old patterns is that the improvement of the condition appears to be too slow. People are not patient enough, so I can suggest one more specific method for quickly improving the condition of the blood.

The Final Weapon

After eating a pure vegetarian diet for more than six months, if your condition does not change significantly, you can try to attack the causative microbes by using salt; this is the final weapon. Salt is a poison for microbes, but makes our body cells stronger. In this case use only good quality natural salt with all its minerals, not refined salt. This is not dangerous for blood pressure or kidney trouble if truly you have not eaten any animal food for more than six months. Very slowly increase the intake of salt in cooked foods. You might feel slightly increased body heat, but this is not fever. Don't increase your liquid intake. Strong people can shower many times a day, and taking a cold bath is also good. This can help relieve a feeling of thirst. Weaker people and those who feel this is too risky shouldn't try it. For them, it is important to patiently accept a longer recovery period.

Take approximately ten grams of salt per day for one week, fifteen grams a day for the next week, then 20 grams, 25 grams, and finally 30 grams. This is the maximum; you don't need more than this and also it is difficult to take.

If you combine salt and oil, such as sauteed vegetables with sesame oil and salt, you won't notice the salt as much. This also helps to avoid thirst. If it is still difficult to continue to take salty food, you can quit at any time and see if anything has changed in your body. If you feel better but haven't recovered, you can try once more. However, strictly prohibit yourself from suddenly drinking a large amount of water even if you feel very thirsty; slowly take water sip by sip over twenty to thirty minutes. Some people cannot tolerate a sudden change, even if it is just plain water.

Health Is Happiness

Many will discover happiness in making a recovery through the natural methods described in this book. Even though some foods are restricted, there are still many things you can eat. As you get better, you become physically more active, your thinking is clearer, you feel good, and it is not difficult for you to continue a natural diet. We don't know the real meaning of life without experiencing suffering. The greatest suffering gives the greatest feeling of happiness. Our world is wonderful. Just living in this world is marvelous. Recovery from the greatest illness is real rebirth and brings true enlightenment. You may discover a new life. This is more powerful than ten thousand words of the greatest philosophers; money, gold, and diamonds are nothing in comparison.

All the steps to health and happiness you must take yourself. You can ask your physician's opinion and you can take medical tests, but you are the one who must take action.

If your medical tests show that your condition is now normal, you can begin to eat any kind of food, but in the beginning very carefully, always paying attention to your physical condition. If you feel anything is wrong, you can understand the problem. You will know your body's condition from your experience. It is said that the AIDS virus can be dormant for twenty or thirty years, but even if some symptoms emerged thirty years later, you would know the cause and how to handle it. You can avoid infections for the rest of your life.

Pneumocystis carinii pneumonia

The most prevalent of the opportunistic AIDS infections is *Pneumocystis carinii* pneumonia (PCP). More than 60 percent of AIDS patients have this infection. It is a new and rare form of pneumonia. In the past few decades this disease has become widespread, although it is seen almost exclusively among immuno-suppressed patients who have had organ transplants or among newborn babies whose immune systems have not yet matured.

Pneumonia is not a disease, but is just a syndrome. Many different microbes cause this trouble and among the other causes are toxic gases such as chlorine. Pneumonia was once a dreaded disease with a high mortality rate, but after the appearance of antibiotics and other drugs, the classic form of pneumonia (caused by bacteria and called labor pneumonia) almost disappeared. But now, new forms of pneumonia caused by viruses are increasing. AIDS pneumonia is said to be caused by a protozoa, a kind of parasite.

The parasite *Pneumocystis carinii* was first observed by the Brazilian microbiologist Carlos Chagas in the lung of a guinea pig in 1909. In the following year Chagas' colleague, A. Carinii, found the same parasite in the lungs of rats. The first case recorded in America was that of a baby who died in a Wisconsin hospital in 1955 from complications resulting from an interstitial plasma cell pneumonia.

Many researchers believe that *Pneumocystis carinii* pneumonia is caused by a parasite. As to transmission routes, many scientists say that parasites travel through the air from the expirations of sick people, while others maintain that insects carry the disease. No one seems to believe that this disease is transmitted through sexual contact. However, any kind of bodily contact with an infected party can transmit the disease to one who suffers from a weakened immune system. This parasite mainly attacks the lungs and sometimes the brain and nervous system. By consuming too much sugar and honey people have weakened their brain and their immune systems, thus exposing the lungs and brain to infection. Brazil is the largest producer of honey and the second largest producer of sugar in the world, and PCP was discovered in Brazil; these facts lend credibility to this hypothesis.

The bodies of babies who died from classic *Pneumocystis carinii* pneumonia were covered all over with purplish or bluish marks. People were horrified to see such an unusual color, but on several occasions I have seen the same bluish marks on the bodies of young boys who died of leukemia. Excess sugar consumption is also an important co-factor in leukemia; the mothers ate sugar during pregnancy and fed their babies candies, cakes, and so on. To me the bluish lesions on the skin are the same color as sugar cane. *Pneumocystis carinii* pneumonia is the most common AIDS-related disease in babies and children.

Pregnant women should not eat sweets, as the fetus is fed by the mother's nutrition. And since the baby's nutrition comes from mother's milk, breast-feeding mothers should eat in the way described in the next section on curing PCP. Again, the main causative co-factor in PCP is excess sugar. If breast milk is insufficient and cow's or goat's milk can be used, then be sure not to add any sugar or lactose in amounts more than two grams per one hundred milliliters.

Treating PCP

In the event of *Pneumocystis carinii* pneumonia, all sugars and honey should be strictly avoided; even one gram is harmful. These are not essential foods for life. Avoid all kinds of high-sugar-content foods including corn syrup, maple syrup, rice syrup, apple juice, orange juice, etc. Even fruits, especially dried fruits such as raisins, dates, figs, bananas, and so on, are not safe and should be avoided as much as possible. If these restrictions seem too harsh, then think of the hundreds of varieties of other foods among grains, beans, seeds, nuts, and vegetables that are available to you and are tasty to the palate and good for your health.

Some people have Kaposi's sarcoma and *Pneumocystis carinii* pneumonia at the same time. This happens to those who eat a lot of meat as well as excessive amounts of sweets. In all cases, these same dietary suggestions are recommended.

Unsafe Solutions

It seems that even x-ray examinations are not entirely safe, especially for an immuno-suppressed patient. It is well known that after x-rays began to be used for diagnosis an ionizing radiation produced severe irritation on the surface of the skin among technicians. Those who worked with x-rays began to look like their bodies were decaying, a condition that was later identified as carcinomic. This is similar to the atom bombs that were dropped on Hiroshima and Nagasaki and that produced a radiation that led to leukemia in many of the casualties.

In April of 1981 a homosexual male was admitted into a San Francisco hospital. He had always been healthy except for bouts of hepatitis and syphilis many years before, but recently he had been complaining of fever and diarrhea.

The first x-rays taken showed his condition to be normal, but three days later he experienced difficulty in breathing and developed a cough. A second set of x-rays showed infiltration by pneumonia. His breathing and coughing became worse. Five days later a piece of his lung was removed for a biopsy. The pathologist was amazed to discover that the lung tissue was severely infected with a protozoan parasite (*Pneumocystis carinii*). His condition failed to improve and it was discovered that he also had a yeast infection (*Candida albicans*). About three months later he died in the hospital.

In retrospect, it is obvious that this patient suffered from AIDS, but the question that needs to be raised is whether or not diagnostic x-rays are a safe procedure in cases of lung disease, especially for an immuno-suppressed patient. We need to ask why the first x-rays showed a normal condition. If this was a mistake, then the radiologist was the one responsible for worsening the patient's condition. It is hard to believe that x-ray examinations are not accurate.

Also, there are no chemical drugs available that are known to be absolutely safe, especially in regard to their effect on the brain. Many anti-cancer drugs, antibiotics, anesthetics, and hypnotic drugs lead to immune suppression. All the more reason why one should not experiment with drugs.

Three to five hundred years ago natural herbs and other organic materials were used pharmaceutically. Today we know that natural quinine is much safer in treating malaria than are synthetic chemical drugs. Vitamin C is a good treatment for cases of Kaposi's sarcoma, but large doses of vitamin C are harmful for *pneumocystis carinii* pneumonia patients. These and many other natural remedies can and should be tested.

Some Japanese doctors tested nine people who tested positive for AIDS with traditional herbal teas. Nihon Keizai Shinbun, one of the largest newspapers in Japan, reported on the work of Dr. Michio Fujimaki, professor of Tokyo School of Medicine, and his colleagues in the April 21, 1987 issue. For a three month trial period they administered Minor (Small) Saikoto to five patients and ginseng herb teas to four patients who were infected with the AIDS virus, but had not yet developed symptoms. Already other researchers had reported that Minor Saikoto strengthens the weakened immune system.

Seven of the nine patients increased their white blood cell count and improved their condition, especially those taking the ginseng herb tea. Blood tests showed that one patient's helper T-cell count had increased from four hundred to eight hundred per milliliter(the norm among healthy people is about fifteen hundred to two thousand), and some of them doubled their natural killer-cells. Several synthetic drugs which were expected to cure AIDS were tested by these doctors on other patients as a control group but no improvement was observed.

These teas have been used in East Asian countries for at least two thousand years, have been tested on countless people, and are considered to be absolutely safe.

This data is derived from too small a sample to prove the effect of herb teas on AIDS patients. We have to wait for further testing. But I don't oppose trying any natural remedy that may help to shorten the recovery time, as the present situation is so urgent. An Oriental herb store can combine the ingredients, as listed in the footnote, for you.[2]

The Root of Disease

Toxic waste materials from meat-eating accumulate quickly and cause disease but are also rapidly excreted and the recovery is quick. Not so for the bad effects of sugar-eating. If one has been eating sugar for ten to twenty years, the lungs and the brain are weaker and more susceptible to disease. This process is very slow and difficult to detect by way of medical tests. So once the disease has appeared, the root is already ten to twenty years deep and the recovery is also very slow. *Pneumocystis carinii* pneumonia patients should thus be very patient.

Your health condition improves very slowly, step by step. The symptoms may disappear within one year, but to rebuild a strong body and a strong immune system you may need seven years or longer. If not, relapse is likely. I know many people want a quick recovery – if possible, an instant recovery. It is possible to speed up the recovery process, but a good understanding of the effects of food – especially animal foods, sugar, and processed foods – is necessary. Be especially careful when visiting your relatives or good friends. They often serve cakes, candies, soft drinks, etc., as an expression of love. Don't take any of them if you are diagnosed with AIDS.

It is well known that a relapse of the AIDS infection always happens, but the reason is unknown. However, I believe this is almost always caused by eating habits. A relapse concerns me more than slow improvement. Eat very carefully until all medical tests show a normal condition. Even if the seven-year recovery process becomes ten years or more, still it is better to be vigorous and to enjoy your life. If you can resolve the right amount of salt as discussed in the salt chapter, and if you chew your food well, the recovery process will be much shorter. Food is a subject of study for your whole life.

Other Opportunistic Infections

Candida albicans is a fairly common condition known as thrush, or yeast infection, caused by a kind of fungus. In the past it was mainly a women's trouble that grew in the more humid parts of the body. The main symptoms were feelings of itchiness, vicious discharge, and sometimes pain. But now this has spread to other parts of the body, including the mouth, eyes, throat, and even inside the body in the digestive tract, lungs, brain, and nervous system.

In his popular book *The Yeast Connection*, Dr. William G. Crook states that eating sugar and the use of penicillin and other antibiotics causes *Candida*. No sugar and no antibiotics are his most important points. He also recommends no bread, cheese, or any fermented foods, such as wine, other alcoholic drinks, or vinegar. Mushrooms should be avoided because they are a kind of fungi. In addition, processed meats such as hot dogs, corned beef, pastrami, etc., are on his not-to-eat list.

However, beneficial fungi are very important for our life and health. There are many kinds of fungi that work together and help us stay healthy. I already mentioned the abstraction from shiitake mushrooms of an interferon-inducing substance. As far as bread is concerned, the yeast in bread is different from the *Candida* yeast. White bread, full of sugar and chemicals and devoid of minerals, should be avoided, but whole wheat bread without sugar or honey can be eaten. (However, commercial baker's yeast is grown with sugar, so naturally-risen bread is recommended.)

Sugar and antibiotics are the most powerful enemies. You need to remember that sugar is the best nutrition for unfriendly fungi and that they are extremely resistant against acid. Acids in the blood support fungal activity. Therefore, the blood pH should be kept at about 7.4. This optimal condition is most important for all diseases.

Once fungi invade the brain, curing is difficult. But before this final stage and especially if the problem is only on the skin or in the mucous membranes, the fungi can be controlled within one month.

For all other opportunistic infections, even though they are caused by various microbes and occur in different parts of the body, still the main co-factors are always the same: too much acid and not enough electrolytes in the blood. This includes herpes simplex, genital herpes, cytomeglovirus, and hepatitis A and B, all caused by viruses and strongly related to simultaneous heavy meat- and sugar-eating. By eating mainly grains and vegetables you can change the quality of your blood, prevent constipation and diarrhea, and always maintain a good condition of the digestive organs. These concerns are controlled by your will and your care. As a result, the proper functioning of your brain, nervous system, organs, glands, and all parts of your body follows without conscious effort. Recovery is possible.

Epilogue

Part 1: Magic Pills

After writing this book, I read an interesting book called *Miracle Cure: Organic Germanium* by Dr. Kazukiko Asai.[1] He is not a medical doctor or a doctor of science but his research was scientific enough that he was elected as a member of the New York Academy of Science in 1975. The effectiveness of his synthetic organic germanium treatments has been verified by medical investigation.

The discovery of germanium is rather new, only about a hundred years old; it is known as a rare element with an atomic number of thirty-two. For about sixty years, germanium received little attention. However, in 1948 it came to be utilized for its semiconducting characteristics and suddenly began to play a major role in the development of modern civilization within the field of electronics. It is the main component in transistors and diodes used in radios, televisions, and many other electrical apparatuses.

Trace amounts of germanium seem essential for growing plants. Many plants contain germanium and large amounts can be found in ginseng and many traditional Chinese herbs. Among common foods, garlic contains the largest amount. Certain kinds of mushrooms, comfrey, and aloe also contain a good amount of germanium. These sources are all organic in form and are useful for our body.

Organic germanium increases the oxygen supply in the body, enables the body cells to take more oxygen and become more active, and creates better metabolism. Doctors assisting Asai discovered that even cancer cells can return to normal when they accept enough oxygen from the blood. Asai succeeded in synthesizing organic germanium from inorganic substances. He emphasized that this organic germanium is not a chemical drug, but rather it is a kind of food. No prescription is needed and no harmful side-effects are reported, and it is safe to use in large doses. Many tests show, more or less, the same good effects, yet he does not say that all sick people will be cured because for many the treatment is already too late. Also, he recommended a well-balanced diet with much alkaline-forming food. He determined sugar to be an acid-forming food and thus his dietary recommendations are very similar to mine.

In reading this book, I wondered why Dr. Asai didn't try his organic germanium treatment on AIDS patients, especially since he is a member of the New York Academy of Science. Soon after, I visited with the publisher of the book and asked about this; it was then I learned that he unfortunately died a few years ago. His germanium is in too much demand for the short supply and is not available to anyone except those who obtain a certificate from the doctors at his clinic.[2] Some health practitioners in California are recommending organic germanium for AIDS patients, but they are using germanium imported from Taiwan and elsewhere. These are adulterated forms of Asai's formula and seem less effective.

The news was disappointing, but I continued to think about this treatment for several days. Our ancestors didn't have any kind of magic pills. Or did they?

Yes, they did. Of course the remedies were not in pill form, but they were the same as magic pills. Many kinds of wine have been thought of as medicine by many different peoples and is the oldest panacea in the world. Even today, many tonics have wine as a base. Salt also has been used as medicine by primitive people. Garlic was used as medicine across the ancient world from Rome to China. Green tea has been used as medicine in Asia. In the seventeenth century, the French and English used coffee as a panacea for anything from sore throats to smallpox. A newer panacea for the Europeans is Korean ginseng. Penicillin is another kind of panacea, or magic pill.

But today, all of them have lost their good reputation and with some, harmful side-effects have been reported. No magic pill exists in the world. Whatever you try, if you use the panacea for a long time, the good effect decreases gradually and finally it loses its effectiveness because the body develops a tolerance. So, it is useless to go to Japan to try organic germanium as a test.

Gautama Buddha taught that nothing is reliable except yourself – not even your children, your spouse, relatives, or friends. Money, gold, diamonds, property, etc., are not helpful. Everything depends on your understanding, self-training, and self-establishment.

This is right. I have to establish my health by myself and you have to establish your health by yourself.

Part 2: About Macrobiotics

Recently I found some encouraging news about AIDS. In fact, the only good news is that now some people recognize that the best preventive measure for AIDS is macrobiotics. The following news comes from New York and Boston where macrobiotic people are teaching their diet to groups of AIDS patients. I quote from the *East West* magazine of September 1986:

> Dr. Martha Cottrell, Director of Student Health at the Fashion Institute of Technology in New York and active with the macrobiotic AIDS group, is a bit more enthusiastic. Currently working on a book about AIDS and macrobiotics, Cottrell says, "The data in the study are absolutely unique. With every other therapy tested, the downward trend in the parameters of blood quality continues unabated. For the first time we have a sign that the decline in the immune function of the body can be stopped and perhaps even reversed."
>
> The positive effects of the macrobiotic approach are discernible not only in the blood analyses. According to observers and to the participants themselves the general physical, emotional, and psychological health of the macrobiotic men is significantly better than that of AIDS patients

receiving other treatments. . . .

Elinor N. Levy, Ph.D., an associate professor in biology at the Boston University School of Medicine, comments that "the men in the study seem to enjoy a quality of life, rare if not unknown, among other men with AIDS. We are hoping to add a psychological component to our testing." "These men," observes Cottrell, "are active. They are working. They are leading normal lives. They meet weekly in support groups to encourage, help, and advise each other. They are optimistic about the future. As a group they are totally distinct from most other AIDS patients who are usually chronically tired and ill, who cannot work, and who are consumed with a feeling of powerlessness and despair." . . .

Three years ago Max DiCorcia was diagnosed as having AIDS and Kaposi's sarcoma, a skin lesion often accompanying the syndrome. A designer and professional cook who has been macrobiotic for about two years, he says, "If anything, I have too much energy. I am very busy in my work. I swim every day. I go out dancing twice a week. I live a typical New York life. Plus I have really come to terms with the illness. I feel that I understand it and that ultimately I am in control. And I see a similar attitude in my macrobiotic friends. Their whole emotional tenor is just very positive." . . .

One participant in the study comments, "Becoming macrobiotic was the hardest thing I ever did. I had to change everything – how I thought, how I ate, how I lived. First I had to take responsibility for my illness. I couldn't think of myself as just an innocent victim any longer. Then I had to give up all the foods I really enjoyed – cheese, ice cream, pastries, coffee, not to mention alcohol and other drugs. I already had given up sex because of the illness, so all together most of my playthings in life were taken away. I had to go from being completely self-indulgent to being a semi-ascetic; from Hugh Hefner to St. Francis."

In another paper the famous immunologist and AIDS researcher, Anthony S. Fauci, M.D. (National Institute of Health, Bethesda, Maryland) says, "Macrobiotics could help prevent the onset of AIDS." If this is the only possible means of AIDS prevention, then why doesn't the Federal Government adopt macrobiotics and publicize it?

I know the reason and it is one based on a misunderstanding of macrobiotics, as we can see in this example, taken from one of the authoritative textbooks on nutrition in this country, *Nutrition and Diet Therapy,* by Sue Rodwell Williams: "Zen macrobiotics eat only brown rice and herb tea. This is done to achieve a perfect balance of yin and yang in order to fend off disease."[3]

This statement is in error. No macrobiotic teacher recommends eating just brown rice and herb tea. Of course, the book was written by someone who does not know macrobiotics, but many people hold this same attitude.

Look in any macrobiotic cookbook such as *The Dō of Cooking* by Cornellia Aihara (George Ohsawa Macrobiotic Foundation) and you will find a wide variety of foods. The origins of macrobiotics came from ancient Zen temples, but now it is separate from religion and is taught as a way of life to gain health and happiness by using natural foods. Already many macrobiotic books have been published in English and are available in health food stores and in some bookstores. Some of the books recommend strict limitations on certain foods for sick people, but food recommendations are always varied according to one's health condition and environment. If you go to the polar region and eat meat like the Eskimos, or if you go to the tropics and eat native fruits such as bananas or pineapples, this is still a macrobiotic approach. True macrobiotic followers are cosmopolitans. The ideal condition is to be free from any and all kinds of bondage, including a strict adherence to any specific diet or food.

But there are problems as evidenced by the following food recommendations of macrobiotic teachers:

Principal food: brown rice, other whole grains, and miso
  soup.
Vegetables: mainly root vegetables, some leaf, stem, or
  flower vegetables.
Pickles: umeboshi, daikon, and others.
Seasoning: salt, miso, soy sauce (tamari), sesame and other
  vegetable oils.
Beans, nuts, seeds: small quantities of certain kinds.
Beverages: Ohsawa coffee (grain beverage), bancha tea, mu
  tea, kokkoh.
Foods to avoid: sugar, red meats, refined foods, highly
  processed foods, tomatoes, potatoes, eggplants, avo-
  cado, asparagus, peanuts, mushrooms (and some
  books list many more).

This is a good diet for the Japanese, but it is not the best for
Americans. Americans should eat local foods; this is true macrobiotics. We have thousands of varieties of foods such as whole corn,
whole wheat bread, locally grown barley, oats, rye, buckwheat,
beans, seeds, nuts, vegetables, and so on. All of them are good.
Local products are always the most suitable and the prices are the
lowest. I repeat: don't eat imported food.

Like all the other original macrobiotic teachers, I learned
macrobiotics from George Ohsawa. However, I have found the
understanding of each to be greatly different. Almost forty years
ago George Ohsawa came to New York and started teaching. At
that time miso, tamari, and other important foods were not available in this country, so he recommended that people buy from Japan
temporarily and soon he made a plan for building a food factory in
California. He had already established a factory in Belgium for
Europeans. But, unfortunately, he died before he realized this plan
for Americans.

Since arriving in this country, I have taught production of special foods such as miso-making at home, soy sauce production, and
how to clean crude sea salt to use for food production. The California

apricot is similar to the Japanese ume plum, so I began making American umeboshi (pickled plums) out of these apricots. These foods are important for vegetarians who don't eat meat. They are high in protein and are rich in amino acids. Umeboshi provides a good amount of citric acid and is rich in potassium, iron, and other nutrients; salt is added and the apricots are pickled with perilla (shiso or chiso) leaves in order to make mineral balance.

But why do we need any specific food? The reason is that miso and soy sauce (tamari) are important sources of protein (amino acids). Our basic foods are of plant origin and as vegetarians we need such kinds of foods, especially if we have any trouble related to malnutrition. Still, these particular foods are not essential. If miso and soy sauce are not available you can find a good substitute such as well-cooked beans with seaweeds. Already some of my students have started food production businesses in this country, but their distribution is still very small. One of the largest American canned soup makers plans to build a huge miso factory in New Jersey, but this has not been accomplished yet. After the Chernobyl nuclear accident, miso soup became suddenly popular in Europe as an anti-radiation food, probably from the experience of Dr. Akizuki in Nagasaki (see page 6). Japanese miso is made nearly 100 percent from American soybeans. Many makers use soybean meal but I strongly oppose this practice. With this situation, who can recommend millions of Americans to eat miso soup every day? Miso should be made in this country using whole soybeans.

I have not written about macrobiotic principles or yin and yang, but if you know a little about macrobiotics, you already know that my dietary recommendations are different from other teachers. For example, I do not say not to eat tomatoes, potatoes, spinach, asparagus, etc. But my suggestions on food selection, quantity, preparation, and so forth are based on the principles of yin and yang, although to avoid needless confusion I have not used such terms. If the produce is local, any kind is good. Some foods have strong characteristics and flavors and require special cooking methods, and in these cases it is wise to learn from the traditional preparations.

The main purpose of macrobiotics is not the healing of disease, but rather the furthering of everyone's happiness. However, as a result of eating a good diet, we can expect recovery from disease. Giving advice to sick people tests our understanding; if our understanding is good we can expect a better result. After you have reestablished your own health, you can give advice to your family, relatives, and friends. These people can spread the understanding to others after they have reestablished their health. I have learned many things from traditional Oriental medicine, macrobiotic principles, herbal teas, and acupuncture. I have been following the diet described here for more than fifty years. An unexpected thing has happened to me: giving advice to sick people has become my business. Evidently, our society needs such a counselor. Whether my job is described as natural hygienist, nutritionist, dietary adviser, or even quackery by the doctors, many things now show that macrobiotics is right.

Since Dr. Sagen Ishizuka started teaching modern macrobiotics in Japan almost a hundred years ago, we have been talking about the same things. The body needs high fever so don't remove it unless it gets to a dangerous state. Pain is good as part of the body's healing process, so it is not good to take pain-killers. We need bulky foods such as dietary fiber. Don't eat sugar; sugar is harmful. Excess meat-eating causes many troubles. High-nutrition foods are questionable, especially if they are refined.

Today, scientific medicine is developing with great velocity and many medical theories have changed. Macrobiotics has not needed to change so much. However, I have changed a few things because I have always needed to learn from new medical and nutritional research in order to communicate with sick people. For example, Dr. Ishizuka's discovery was that sodium and potassium were the most important elements for body balancing and that the ratio should be five parts potassium to one part sodium. In modern nutritional theory this is only one body balancing ratio. Others such as calcium and phosphorus also need to be maintained. My idea is to include and balance the sums of all the positive and negative electrical forces in the body.

Now, we are facing the problem of AIDS. Some researchers fear that our entire population may be infected with the AIDS virus in the near future. I don't think this will happen, but so many other difficult diseases are increasing. It is time for all Americans to change their diets. I am trying to open the door to macrobiotics for everyone. This is necessary not only for AIDS prevention, but also at the same time to keep everyone free from infectious diseases.

After reading this book, watch people's diets carefully. Who are prone to AIDS and who are weak against other infections? However, we don't have five or ten years to wait. The problem is so urgent that you have to decide right now. Accept my opinion and practice it or not, everything is depending on your decision. But nature is always dividing us strictly and inevitably into two groups – life or death.

If you have questions, please reread this book and try to discover the answers by yourself. If mistakes or omissions are found, they will be corrected in forthcoming editions. If any public institution or hospital treating many AIDS patients wants to try my ideas, I will be glad to go and show how my dietary recommendations work. If any large public hospital, school of medicine, state or federal government, foreign country, or large newspaper asks me questions through my publisher, I will try to respond.

Noboru Muramoto
March 1988

Symbols

ACTH	adrenocorticotrophic hormone
AIDS	aquired immune deficiency syndrome
ARC	AIDS-related complex
ARV	AIDS-associated retrovirus
AZT	azidothimidine
C	carbon
Ca	calcium
CAT	computerized axial tomography
CDC	Centers for Disease Control
CMV	cytomegalovirus
CO_2	carbon dioxide
CO	carbon monoxide
DNA	deoxyribonucleic acid
EBV	Epstein-Barr virus
ELISA	enzyme-linked immunosorbent assay
F or f	female
°F	degrees Farenheit
FDA	Food and Drug Administration
Fe	iron
H	hydrogen
HD	Hansen's Disease
H_2O	water

HIV	human immune-deficiency virus
HTLV-I	human T-cell leukemia virus, type one
HTLV-III	human T-cell lymphotropic virus, type three
IF	Interferon
IL	Interleukin
JAMA	Journal of the American Medical Association
K	potassium (kalium)
KS	Kaposi's sarcoma
LAV	lymphadenopathy-associated virus
M or m	male
M.D.	medical doctor
Mg	magnesium
mg	milligram
MSG	monosodium-glutamate
MS	multiple sclerosis
mv	millivolt
N	nitrogen
Na	sodium (natrium)
NaCl	sodium chloride
NCL	National Cancer Institute
NH_3	ammonia
NIH	National Institute of Health
NO_2	nitrite
NO_3	nitrate
NS	nervous system
O	oxygen
OI	opportunistic infection

P	phosphorus
PCP	*Pneumocystis carinii* pneumonia
PET	positron emission tomography
pH	measure of acidity and alkalinity
ppm	parts per million
PSNS	parasympathetic nervous system
Retro	reverse transciptase containing oncogenic virus
RNA	ribonucleic acid
S	sulfur
SNS	sympathetic nervous system
STD	sexually transmitted disease
TB	tuberculosis
USDA	United States Department of Agriculture
v	vitamin
WHO	World Health Organization

Notes

Chapter 1. AIDS Outlook

1. See Robert B. Belshe, *Textbook of Human Virology* (Littleton: PSG Publishing Co., 1984).

2. R.J. Cohen and others in *The New England Journal of Medicine* (June 16, 1983) 308: 1475-6 and Alan Cantwell Jr., M.D., *AIDS: The Mystery and the Solution* (Los Angeles: Aries Rising Press, 1983), 132-151.

3. Alan Fauci Jr., M.D. and H. Clifford Lane, "Etiology of the Acquired Immunodeficiency Syndrome," in John I. Gallin, M.D. and Anthony S. Fauci, M.D., eds., *Acquired Immunodeficiency Syndrome (AIDS) Advances in Host Defense Mechanisms, Vol. 5* (New York: Raven Press, 1985), 30.

4. Alice Lorraine Smith, *Principles of Microbiology* (St. Louis: Times Mirror/ Mosby College Publishing, 1984), 294.

5. Gallin, *Acquired Immunodeficiency Syndrome (AIDS)*, 31.

6. Peter Ebbesen and others, *AIDS* (Philadelphia: W.B. Saunders and Co., 1984), 19.

7. James I. Slaff and John K. Brubaker, *The AIDS Epidemic* (New York: Warner Books, 1985), 169.

8. Joseph A. Kovacs and Henry Masur, "Treatment of Opportunistic Infections," in Ebbesen, *AIDS*, 158.

9. Slaff, *AIDS Epidemic*, 84.

10. Roderick E. McGrew, *Encyclopedia of Medical History* (New York: McGraw-Hill Book Company, 1985), 303.

11. Dennia Altman, *AIDS in the Mind of America* (New York: Anchor Press/ Doubleday, 1986), 148.

12. James R. Allen and James W. Curran, "Epidemiology of the Acquired Immunodeficiency Syndrome," in Gallin, *Acquired Immunodeficiency Syndrome (AIDS)*, 11.

13. Slaff, *AIDS Epidemic*, 157-8.

14. Ebbesen, *AIDS*, 61-2.

15. Alan Cantwell Jr., M.D., *AIDS: The Mystery and the Solution* (Los Angeles: Aries Rising Press, 1983), 97.

Chapter 2. Plagues and Epidemics

1. McGrew, *Encyclopedia of Medical History*, 339.

2. Frances Winwal, *The Decameron of Giovanni Boccaccio* (New York: The Modern Library, 1955), xxiv-xxix.

3. Yoichiro Murakami, *Plague* (Tokyo: Iwanami Publishing Company, 1983). [In Japanese.]

4. From Murakami, *Plague*.

Chapter 3. The Meat-Eater's Body

1. Anthony Smith, *The Body* (New York: Viking-Penguin, Inc., 1986), 95.

2. See Alvin E. Friedman-Kien, M.D. and Linda J. Laubenstein, eds., *AIDS: The Epidemic of Kaposi's Sarcoma and Opportunistic Infections* (New York: Masson Publishing USA, 1983), Chapter 4.

3. See Margot Joan Fromer, *A Comprehensive and Up-to-Date Investigation of the Causes, Methods of Transmission, Symptoms, and Current Research on AIDS* (New York: Pinnacle Books, 1983).

4. Fromer, *Comprehensive AIDS*, 174.

5. Sue Rodwell Williams, *Nutrition and Diet Therapy* (St. Louis: Times Mirror/Mosby College Publishing, 1985), 255.

6. Alan E. Read and others, eds., *Modern Medicine* (London: Pitman Press, 1984), 264.

7. Bernard Jensen, *Iridology: The Science and Practice of the Healing Arts* (Escondido: Bernard Jensen, Pub., 1982), 232-3.

8. Henry Bieler, M.D., *Food is Your Best Medicine* (New York: Random House, 1965), 190-1.

9. Dr. Jay M. Hoffman, *Hunza* (Escondido: Professional Press Publishing Association, 1973), 185-6.

Chapter 4. Sugar

1. Williams, *Diet Therapy*, 43.

2. Robert S. Boikes and others, *Elements of Chemistry* (New Jersey: Prentice-Hall, 1986), 465.

3. Boikes, *Elements of Chemistry*, 252.

4. John Yudkin, *Sweet and Dangerous* (New York: Bantam, 1973), 157-66.

5. Boikes, *Elements of Chemistry*, 655.

6. William F. Ganong, M.D., *Review of Medical Physiology*, (Los Altos: Lange Medical Publications, 1985), 440.

Chapter 5. Grains

1. *Encyclopedia Britannica* (fifteenth edition), 3:1157.

2. Based on data from *FAO Production Yearbook* (Rome: FAO/UN, 1979), vol. 33.

3. Stephen Mennell, *All Manners of Food* (New York: Basil Blackwell, 1985), 48.

4. Ronald E. Kotzsch, Ph.D., *Macrobiotics: Yesterday and Today* (Tokyo: Japan Publications, 1985), 29.

5. Williams, *Diet Therapy*, 81-95.

6. See Hoffman, *Hunza*.

7. Based on data from *FAO Production Yearbook* (Rome: FAO/UN, 1979), vol. 33.

Chapter 6. Beans, Seeds, and Nuts

1. Audrey Ensminger, *Foods and Nutrition Encyclopedia* (Clovis: Pegus Press, 1983), 1279.

2. Ensminger, *Foods and Nutrition Encyclopedia*, 365.

3. J. I. Rodale, *Prevention Method for Better Health* (Emmaus: Rodale Books, Inc., 1966), 328.

Chapter 7. Vegetables and Fruits

1. Ensminger, *Foods and Nutrition Encyclopedia*, 1974.

2. Data from the Norwegian Seaweed Institute, as reported in *Review of Seaweed Research* (Clemson University: Research Series No. 76, 1966).

3. Adapted from Herman Aihara, *Acid and Alkaline* (Oroville: George Ohsawa Macrobiotic Foundation, 1986), 56.

4. *Encyclopedia Britannica*, 7:37.

5. Based on *Handbook of the Nutritional Contents of Foods*, U.S. Department of Agriculture.

6. Based on *Handbook of the Nutritional Contents of Foods*, U.S. Department of Agriculture.

Chapter 8. Salt

1. Quoted from Rudolf Hauschka, *Nutrition* (London: Rudolf Steiner Press, 1983), 67.

2. *Prevention*, August 1986, 65.

3. Gerhard Schmidt, *The Dynamics of Nutrition* (Wyoming: Bio-Dynamic Literature, 1980), 113ff.

4. Schmidt, *Dynamics of Nutrition*, 113ff.

5. Ensminger, *Foods and Nutrition Encyclopedia*, 1:406 and 2:1513.

6. John D. Kirschman, *Nutrition Almanac* (New York: McGraw-Hill Books, 1984), 169.

7. From *Encyclopedia Britannica* (fifteenth edition).

8. Figures calculated from *Handbook of the Nutritional Contents of Foods*, U.S. Department of Agriculture. Magnesium calculated from *Food and Nutrition Encyclopedia*. Sulfur and Chlorine calculated from *The Chemistry of Man*, Dr. Bernard Jensen.

9. Figures calculated from *Handbook of the Nutritional Contents of Foods*, U.S. Department of Agriculture. Magnesium calculated from *Food and Nutrition Encyclopedia*. Sulfur and Chlorine calculated from *The Chemistry of Man*, Dr. Bernard Jensen.

Chapter 9. Chewing

1. William F. Ganong, M.D., *Review of Medical Physiology* (Los Angeles: Lange Medical Publications, 1985), 399. See also Lennart Nilsson, *The Body Victorious* (New York: Delacorte Press, 1987), 150.

2. Renee Taylor, *Hunza Health Secrets* (New York: Award Books, 1964), 100.

3. William Alexander Dorland, *American Medical Dictionary* (Philadephia: W. B. Saunders and Co., 1981), 971.

Chapter 12. The Immune System

1. Lewis Thomas, *The Youngest Science* (New York: Bantam Books, 1984), 202.

2. Frederick P. Siegal, M.D. and Marta Siegal, M.A., *AIDS: The Medical Mystery* (New York: Grove Press, 1983), 20.

3. Norman Cousins, *Mind as Apothecary* introduced in *Consumers Digest* March/April 1985. from Richard Bergland M.D. of Harvard Medical School.

Chapter 13. The Harmony and Balance of the World

1. William H. McNeill, *Plagues and Peoples* (New York: Anchor Press, 1976), 286.

2. Michael Harner in *Quest for the Past*, ed. by Reader's Digest (New York: Random House, 1984), 279.

Chapter 15. Body Balance and Central Control

1. From Dr. Shiro Kawashima, *Natural Hygiene* (Tokyo: Kodansha International, 1977).

2. Boikes, *Elements of Chemistry*, 252.

Chapter 16. AIDS Symptoms and Strategies

1. Fromer, *Comprehensive AIDS*, 161-2.

2. Gene Antonio, *AIDS Cover-Up?* (Westchester: Ignatius Press, 1986), 89.

3. See Boikes, *Elements of Chemistry*.

4. Joe Henderson, *The Runner's Diet* (Mountain View: Anderson World, Inc., 1978), 111.

5. Tatsuichiro Akizuki, M.D., *Nagasaki 1945* (London: Quartet Books, 1981).

Chapter 17. Full-Blown AIDS

1. *Los Angeles Times*, February 3, 1987.

2. Ginseng herb tea ingredients: 3 grams ginseng; 3 grams licorice; 3 grams jutsu (atractylodes); and 3 grams ginger (or 1 gram dry ginger). Minor (small) saikoto tea ingredients: 5 grams saiko (bupleurum); 4 grams hange (rhizoma pinellia); 3 grams ginseng; 3 grams ogon (scute); 3 grams daiso (jujube fruits); 2 grams licorice; and 1 gram dry ginger.

Epilogue

1. Dr. Kazukiko Asai, *Miracle Cure: Organic Germanium* (Tokyo: Japan Publications, 1980).

2. Organic Germanium Clinic, 6-4-13, Seigo, Setagaya-ku, Tokyo, Japan, phone 03-482-0590.

3. Williams, *Nutrition and Diet Therapy*, 98.

Index